Dental and Maxillofacial Radiology

Dental and Maxillofacial Radiology

James McIvor FDSRCS, FRCR

Senior Lecturer in Radiology, Institute of Dental Surgery, University of London;
Consultant Radiologist, Charing Cross Hospital (Fulham), London, UK

CHURCHILL LIVINGSTONE
EDINBURGH LONDON MELBOURNE AND NEW YORK 1986

CHURCHILL LIVINGSTONE
Medical Division of Longman Group Limited

Distributed in the United States of America by Churchill
Livingstone Inc., 1560 Broadway, New York, N.Y.
10036, and by associated companies, branches and
representatives throughout the world.

First published 1986

ISBN 0 443 03448 6

British Library Cataloguing in Publication Data
McIvor, James
    Dental and maxillofacial radiology.
    1. Maxilla — Diseases 2. Diagnosis, Radioscopic
    I. Title
    617'.520757   RC815

Library of Congress Cataloging in Publication Data
McIvor, James.
    Dental and maxillofacial radiology.

    Bibliography: p.
    Includes index.
    1. Teeth — Radiography. 2. Jaws — Radiography.
    3. Face — Radiography. I. Title. [DNLM: 1. Face —
    radiography. 2. Jaw — radiography. 3. Radiography,
    Dental. WN 230 M478d]
    RK309.M39 1986   617.6'0757   85-12740

Printed and bound in Great Britain by William Clowes
Limited, Beccles and London

Preface

The purpose of this book is to describe and illustrate the radiological abnormalities which result from disease of the teeth and jaws. Most disorders of this region produce changes in calcified tissues which are readily demonstrated by conventional radiography. However, the newer imaging techniques of CT scanning and ultrasound have a valuable role in the assessment of soft tissue masses and malignant tumours and a few examples are therefore included.

Although intended mainly for dental students and practising dental surgeons, it is hoped that this book might also be of value to dental surgeons and radiologists preparing for postgraduate degrees and it is for the benefit of these groups that some rare conditions and a few radiographic and radiological techniques are described in small print.

London, 1986   J.M.

Acknowledgements

I am grateful to Dr J.J. Prior, formerly consultant radiologist at the Eastman Dental Hospital, London for his help and advice in the preparation of this book and to Dr F.L. Ingram, formerly consultant radiologist at the Eastman Dental Hospital, London for access to his collection of radiographs which provided many of the illustrations.

I would like to thank Dr B.E. Kendall, consultant radiologist at the National Hospital for Nervous Diseases, London for Fig. 6.7; Dr T. Doyle, radiologist at the Royal Melbourne Hospital, Australia for Figs 14.3, 14.4; Dr J.E. Boultbee, consultant radiologist at Charing Cross Hospital, London for Figs 15.10B, 15.11B and Dr A.J. Stacey, principal physicist in charge of Medical Physics, Charing Cross Hospital, London for Fig. 1.5.

Finally my thanks are due to Mr A.R. Williams and his colleagues in the Department of Medical Illustration, Charing Cross and Westminster Medical School, London for the care with which they produced photographic prints from the original radiographs, and to my wife, Elizabeth, for typing the manuscript.

Contents

1

Radiographs and other images

PRODUCTION OF RADIOGRAPHS

Radiographs are shadow pictures in black and white. They are produced by passing an X-ray beam through the body and recording the intensity of the attenuated beam on radiographic film, which responds to X-rays in the same way as photographic film responds to light. The silver bromide crystals in the film emulsion which have been in the shadow of radio-opaque structures, such as bones and teeth, are removed by processing and leave the film clear, whereas crystals which have been *sensitised* by radiation remain behind as a black deposit. The result is that radio-opaque tissues cast a white 'shadow' on the dark background of the developed film.

Metallic restorations of amalgam or gold alloys absorb all the energy from the X-ray beam and appear completely white. Calcified structures absorb most of the energy from the beam and appear grey-white.

Enamel, which is the most heavily calcified tissue in the human body (97% calcified inorganic material), is whiter than other calcified tissues such as bone, dentine and cementum which contain approximately 70% calcified inorganic material (Fig. 1.1A, B).

Soft tissues absorb some of the energy from the X-ray beam and appear grey. All soft tissues except fat have the same radio-opacity and produce the same degree of shadowing, but fat is slightly more radiolucent and appears darker. This is of little value in the maxillofacial region, but is of considerable value in abdominal radiology. Air in the buccal cavity and sinuses produces no attenuation of the X-ray beam and appears black.

The *spectrum* on an X-ray film can be summarised as:

WHITE (radio-opaque structures)
   Metallic restorations, e.g. amalgam, gold alloys
   Enamel
   Bone, dentine, cementum and other calcified structures

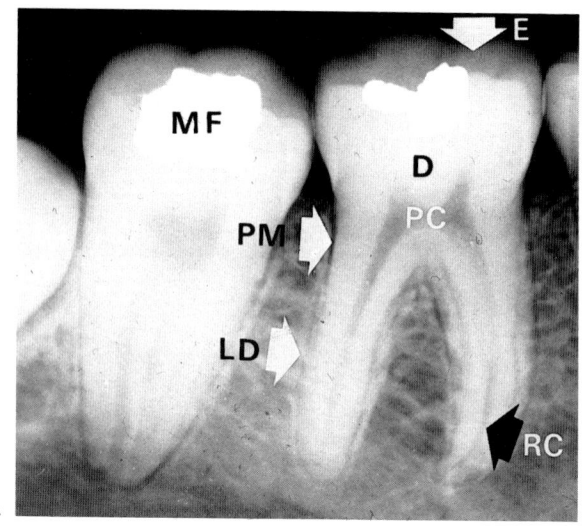

A

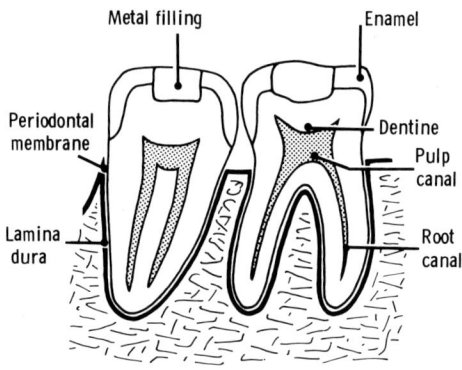

B

Fig. 1.1 A   Labelled radiograph of restored 7̄| and 6̄|. E = Enamel D = Dentine PC = Pulp canal RC = Root canal PM = Periodontal membrane LD = Lamina dura MF = Metallic filling. **B** Line diagram of the radiograph.

GREY
    All soft tissues and fluids, e.g. muscle, cartilage, blood
    except
    Fat

BLACK (radiolucent structures)
    Air

Film cassettes containing intensifying screens, usually crystals of calcium tungstate, make it possible to sensitise an X-ray film with less radiation than is required to sensitise the same film without intensifying screens, as they convert some of the X-rays into visible light to which the film is more sensitive. The advantage is that the patient receives a lower dose of radiation and, in general, this outweighs the disadvantage of a slight loss of resolution. Cassette films with intensifying screens are used for all extra-oral radiography in the maxillo-facial region, but are too bulky for routine intra-oral use.

Non screen dental films are used for most intra-oral radiographs and consist of an X-ray film in a flexible plastic envelope. This resolution is better than the resolution of the same film in a cassette with intensifying screens and this is of particular value in detecting the early changes of dental caries of periodontal disease.

X-rays or *gamma rays* are produced by electrons striking the focal spot of the anode of an X-ray tube. The tube casing, which surrounds the anode, absorbs most of the radiation, but allows a narrow beam, the centre of which is described as the *central ray,* to emerge through a radiolucent window. The intensity of the beam depends on the *inverse square law* and falls by the square of the distance from the focal spot. There is *magnification* on all radiographs as X-rays travel in straight lines and cannot be focussed.

The *exposure factors* required to produce a radiograph are the voltage, current and the time for which they pass through the tube. The units are

kV = kilovolts (1000 volts), usually 60–90

mA = milliampère (1/1000 ampère)

s = seconds

The degree of film blackening produced by a beam of X-rays is directly proportional to the current and time and these units are often combined as milliamp seconds or mA.s. The relationship between blackening and voltage is more complex and is roughly proportional to the square of the voltage.

The exposure time for a radiograph is quite long by normal photographic standards and may exceed 0.5 seconds. Any movement by the patient or X-ray equipment during this period will blur the image and is usually described as *movement blur.*

CEPHALOMETRIC RADIOGRAPHY

The aim of cephalometric radiography is to obtain a radiograph of the facial bones and skull in which the radiographic projection and magnification are standardised and reproducible.

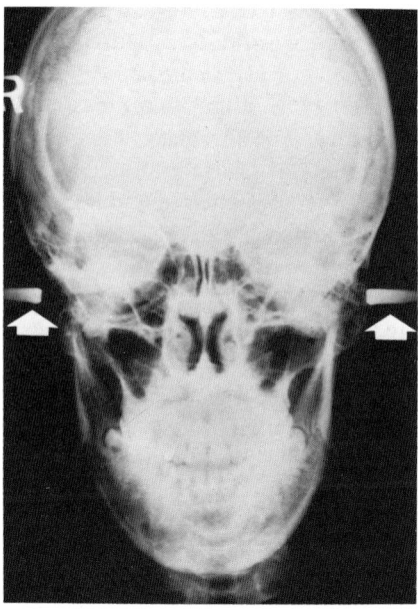

Fig. 1.2 PA cephalostat film showing radio-opaque earplugs (arrowed) in the external auditory meate, which should be completely superimposed on a correctly positioned lateral film.

Cephalometric radiographs are used to assess orthodontic malocclusions and abnormalities of facial development. Techniques are available for obtaining films in lateral and PA projections and in both cases earplugs, attached to hinged arms, are placed in the external auditory meati to immobilise the patient's head (Fig. 1.2). In a correctly positioned lateral film the central ray of the X-ray beam passes through both earplugs and this can be checked on the developed film as the radio-opaque earplugs should be exactly superimposed. There is no general agreement about the magnification which should be present on cephalostat films. Traditionally the distance between the focal spot of the X-ray tube and the film (the film–focus distance or FFD) was 6 feet (1.8 m) and the distance between the mid-line of the skull and the film (the object–film distance) was 5 or 6 inches (130–150 mm), but some modern equipment has a film–focus distance of 5 feet (1.5 m). The advantage of a long film–focus distance is that magnification is kept to a minimum.

A wedge-shaped *aluminium filter* can be used to weaken the beam where it passes through the soft tissues of the face, so that the soft tissue contour can be shown on the same films as the underlying bones.

More elaborate techniques for photographing the patient and superimposing the photographs and the radiographs have been described.[4]

TOMOGRAPHY

A tomogram is an image of a *slice* of tissue.

A *radiographic tomogram* is produced by moving the X-ray tube and film about a fulcrum. Structures which are at the level of the fulcrum have the same relationship to the X-ray tube and film throughout the movement and produce clear shadows, whereas structures above or below the fulcrum produce blurred unrecognisable shadows.

The *thickness* of the slice depends upon the extent and complexity of the movement. For instance, the linear movement through 20° will demonstrate a relatively thick slice of about 1 cm, whereas more complicated circular or hypocycloidal movements can demonstrate slices of 1 mm in thickness.

Tomography has no place in intra-oral radiography as films cannot be moved in the mouth.

The dose of radiation received in the course of a tomographic examination is much higher than the dose for a plain film examination as each tomographic slice exposes the patient to as much radiation as a single plain film and it may be necessary to take five or ten tomographic slices.

All the images produced by *ultrasound* (US) and *computerised tomography* (CT) are tomograms.

PANORAMIC RADIOGRAPHS

Panoramic extra-oral radiographs of the jaws are tomograms in which the slice is curved to conform with the shape of the dental arches. This is usually achieved with a narrow X-ray beam which rotates around the patient's head opposite a special cassette. Modern equipment will usually show both dental arches, the lower parts of the maxillary sinuses, the whole of the mandible and both temporomandibular joints. The disadvantage is that the shape of the slice is fixed and this results in poor definition, particularly in the anterior region, if the dental arches are unusual in shape (Figs 1.3, 1.4).

Intra-oral panoramic dental radiographs are produced by placing one end of a small X-ray tube in the mouth and applying a flexible X-ray film over the maxilla or mandible. The detail is excellent but there is considerable magnification and the field size is smaller than the field

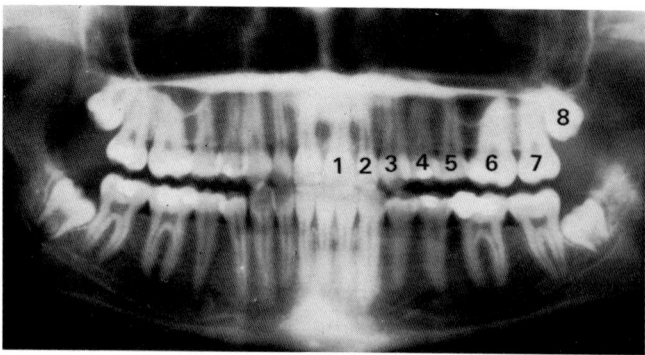

Fig. 1.3   Panoramic radiograph of a normal adult aged 18 years, in which the teeth in the upper left quadrant have been labelled. The third molars are unerupted.

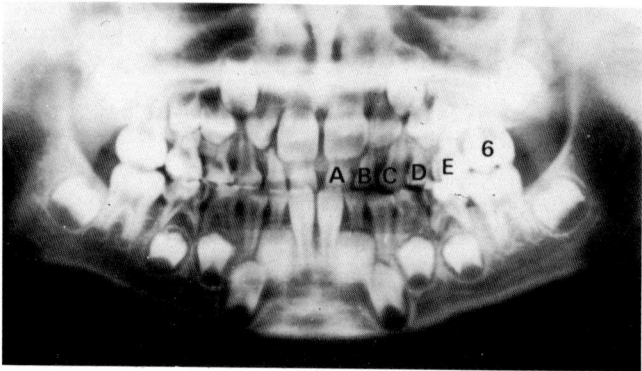

Fig. 1.4   Panoramic radiograph of a normal child aged 6 years, in which the erupted teeth in the upper left quadrant have been labelled.

size of an extra-oral panoramic radiograph. Although much ingenuity has gone into the design of this equipment it has not been widely accepted and is usually regarded as an interesting curiosity.

XERORADIOGRAPHS

A xeroradiograph is produced with conventional X-ray equipment which passes a beam of X-rays through the patient as in conventional radiography. However, the method of recording the image is quite different. The beam falls on an electrostatically charged *selenium plate* in a special cassette and the areas of the plate which are irradiated lose their positive charge. The plate is then dusted with a negatively charged white powder which adheres to the non-irradiated areas, which have retained their positive charge. The powder image is then transferred to a special plasticised paper and fixed.

The image is usually a print, not a transparency and is viewed under direct light. Radio-opaque structures appear white against a dark blue background, as in conventional radiography, but the polarity of the image can be reversed with modern equipment so that the radio-opaque structures appear black or blue-black.

The detail on a xeroradiograph is as good as the detail on a non-screen radiograph and there is the added advantage of *edge enhancement* at tissue interfaces, which improves the visibility of small structures and allows a wide range of tissue densities to be shown on a single picture. This quality is valuable in the maxillofacial region[1] where the structures being visualised range from densely radio-opaque metallic fillings to completely radiolucent air in the buccal cavity and maxillary sinuses (Fig. 1.5).

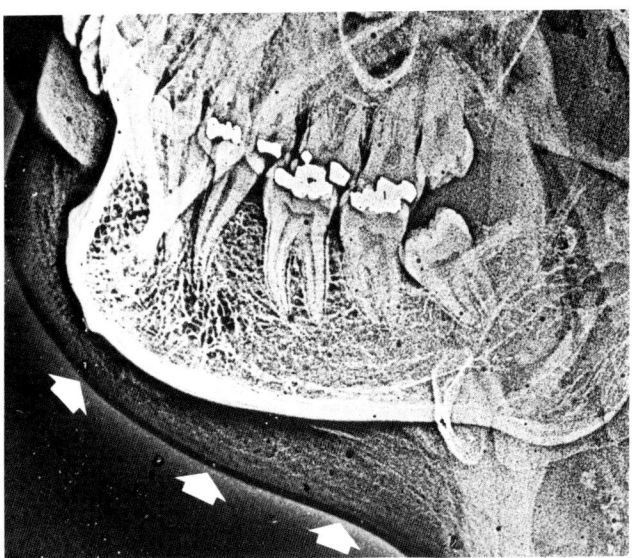

Fig. 1.5 Xeroradiogram of mandible (oblique projection). The metallic fillings and pulp canals of the molar teeth can be readily identified. The trabecular pattern of the mandible is clearer and sharper than on a conventional radiograph and the skin surface (arrowed) is quite well shown, owing to 'edge enhancement'.

The main disadvantage of the technique is that the dose of radiation received by the patient is similar to the dose received when non screen film is used and is therefore higher than the dose received when the image is recorded on radiographic film in a cassette with intensifying screens.

CONTRAST MEDIA

Contrast medium is widely used in general radiology and has a limited place in the maxillofacial region. All contrast media depend upon the iodine or barium atom for radio-opacity. Most *iodine-containing media* are water-soluble or oil-based. Water soluble contrast (e.g. Conray®, Urografin®, Niopam®, Omnipaque®) can be injected directly into veins, arteries and body cavities and is rapidly excreted by the kidneys. Oil-based contrast (e.g. Lipiodol®) is less irritant and more viscous and is used to outline epithelium-lined structures such as the bronchial tree.

Barium contrast media are fine suspensions of barium sulphate and are used for barium swallows and other examinations of the alimentary tract. Barium sulphate is sometimes added to dental cements to render them radio-opaque.

CT SCANNING

Computed tomography (CT) uses X-rays from a high kV tube (120 kV) to produce a *tomographic image* which depends, like a radiograph, on tissue radio-opacity. The X-ray beam passes through the body from different directions and the attenuation or weakening of the beam is measured by a series of detectors. A computer calculates the radio-opacity of each *voxel* of tissue and gives it a *Hounsfield number*. The size of the voxel is approximately 1.5 mm × 1.5 mm × 13 mm, the last being the thickness of the slice, but modern equipment can produce images using a voxel size of less than half this. The image is produced on a TV screen and is subsequently photographed.

The fixed points of the Hounsfield scale are dense bone at +1000, water at zero and air at -1000, and the spectrum can be summarised as follows:

WHITE

+1000	Dense bone
+30–60	Blood clot
+50–70	Most organs and soft tissues
+40–50	Liquid blood
+10–15	Cerebro-spinal fluid

GREY

0	Water
-50–100	Fat

BLACK

-1000	Air

The great advantage of CT over conventional radiography lies in its ability to distinguish between different types of soft tissue and this is of particular value in detecting the spread of malignant tumours.[2,3] It is also possible to obtain the Hounsfield number of any area within the slice and this may assist diagnosis, as some tissues and pathological conditions have characteristic Hounsfield numbers.

The radiation dose is approximately 1 rad (cGy) and is received by each slice of tissue as it is being examined. Although this is higher than the dose received when a single radiograph is taken, it is lower than the dose received during radiographic tomography, as these examinations require multiple slices and each slice exposes the whole thickness of the body to the X-ray beam.

The main disadvantage of CT is the expense.

ULTRASOUND

Ultrasound (US) images are *echo pictures* produced by pulsing a beam of *high frequency ultrasound* (1.5–10 MHz) into the body from a transducer which is applied to the skin surface. High-frequency ultrasound travels through soft tissue at a constant speed, so the source of each echo can be calculated from the time interval between transmitting the pulse and receiving the echo.

The physics of sound reflection is extremely complex but, broadly speaking, strong echoes are produced by organ capsules, the walls of large arteries and veins and some soft tissues, particularly fat. Weaker echoes are produced by small tissue interfaces within organs and by most soft tissues. Fluids, such as blood, and a few soft tissues produce no echoes at all. The image is produced on a TV screen and is subsequently photographed.

The spectrum of an ultrasound picture is complicated and this summary is much simplified:

WHITE (echogenic structures)
   Thick tissue interfaces, e.g. organ capsules, large arteries
   A few soft tissues, particularly fat

GREY
   Most soft tissues

BLACK (transonic structures)
   Fluids, e.g. blood
   A few soft tissues

Most equipment has a frequency of 600 pulses per second, which means that a moving image can be shown on a TV screen by rotating the transducer mechanically, or by using a series of transducers. The moving image is known as a *real time* image.

The image is a *tomogram* and the thickness of the slice is the width of the ultrasound beam which, for practical purposes, is the diameter of the transmitting and receiving transducer.

The advantages of diagnostic ultrasound are that it differentiates between different types of soft tissue in a way that is impossible with conventional radiographs and that it is much cheaper than CT. In addition, there are no harmful biological effects and this accounts for its extensive use in obstetrics. Its main disadvantage is that high-frequency ultrasound is completely absorbed or reflected by *bone* and *gas*, which cast an acoustic shadow. This is a severe limitation in the maxillofacial region, but the technique has a role in the assessment of palpable soft tissue masses such as swollen parotid glands.

REFERENCES

1. Binnie W M, Stacey A J, Davis R, Cawson R A 1975 Applications of xeroradiography in dentistry. Journal of Dentistry 3: 99–104
2. Daniels D L, Rauschning W, Lovas J et al 1983 Pterygo-palatine fossa: computed tomographic studies. Radiology 149: 511–516
3. Doubleday L C, Bao-Shan J, Wallace S 1981 Computed tomography of the infratemporal fossa. Radiology 138: 619–624
4. Fanibunda K B 1983 Photoradiography of facial structures. British Journal of Oral and Maxillofacial Surgery 21: 246–258

2

Caries, peri-apical infection and dental restorations

CARIES

Dental caries is a destructive process which affects the enamel and dentine of erupted or partially erupted teeth. The destructive process commonly begins at irregularities in the occlusal surfaces of molars and pre-molars (pit and fissure caries), or below the contact points of adjacent teeth (interproximal caries).

The earliest radiological change is a small pit in the enamel surface which is difficult or impossible to demonstrate radiographically, but when the carious process has penetrated the enamel and reached the dentine the full-thickness defect can usually be demonstrated on an intra-oral non-screen film (Fig. 2.1). The destruction of dentine progresses much more rapidly than the destruction of enamel as dentine

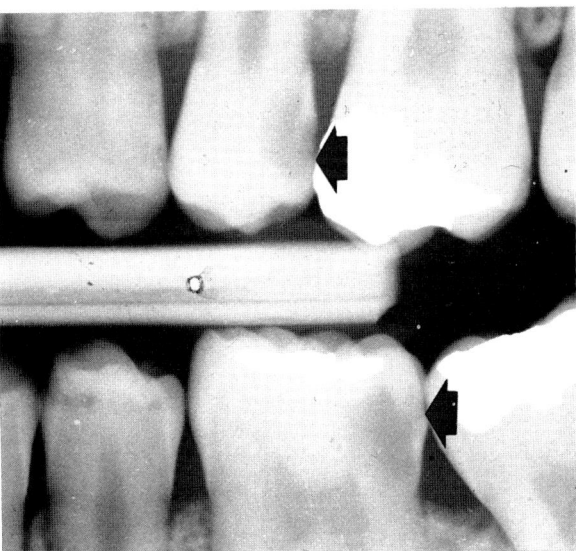

Fig. 2.1 Distal inter proximal caries of 5⌋ and 6⌉ with small defects in the overlying enamel (arrowed).

11

is less heavily calcified and as bacteria will grow along the dentinal tubules if they are still patent. The extent of dentinal destruction is always more extensive than is apparent from a radiograph as the radiolucency of calcified tissues is probably not altered until decalcification exceeds 50% (Fig. 2.2A, B). If unchecked, the process continues until the crown is completely destroyed (Fig. 2.3).

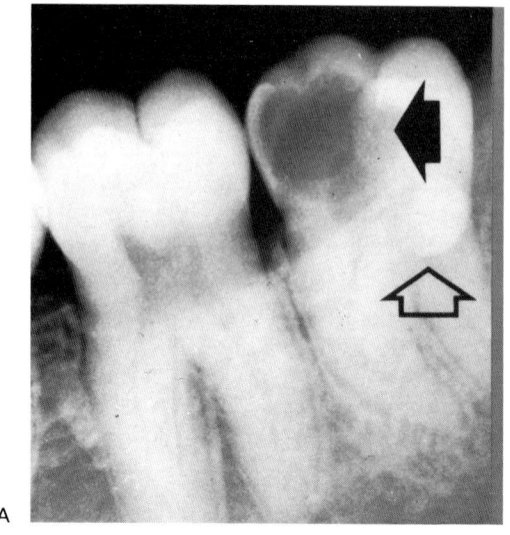

A

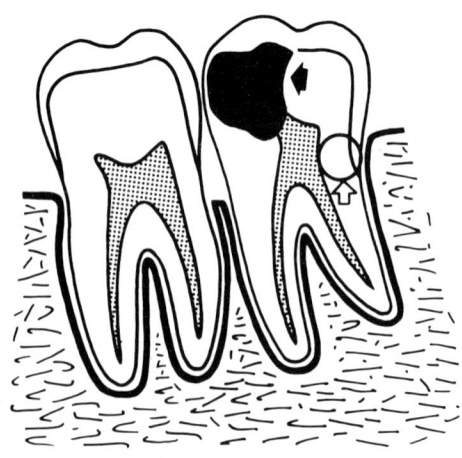

B

Fig. 2.2 A   Advanced occlusal caries of $\overline{8}$ (solid arrow). The defect in the enamel of the occlusal surface if faintly visible. The open arrow points to an enameloma or enamel pearl. **B** Line diagram of the radiograph.

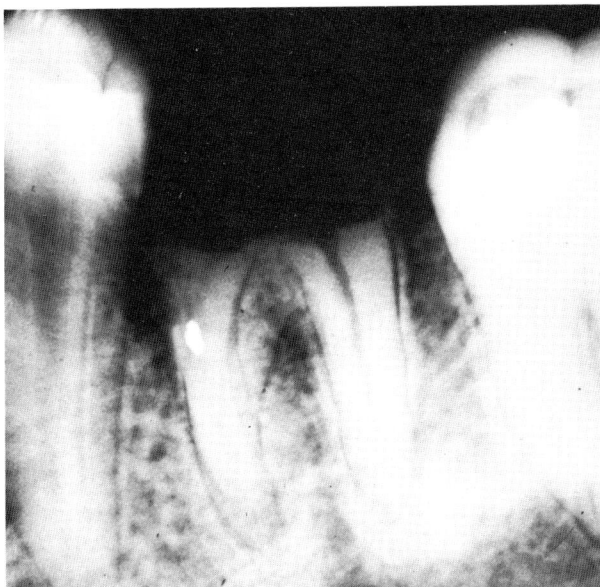

Fig. 2.3 Complete destruction of the crown of ⌐6 due to advanced caries. The metallic opacity overlying the mesial root is a fragment of amalgam in a periodontal pocket.

In partially erupted and abnormally erupted teeth, the carious lesion can begin anywhere and may be detected radiographically before there is any clinical evidence of disease (Fig. 2.4).

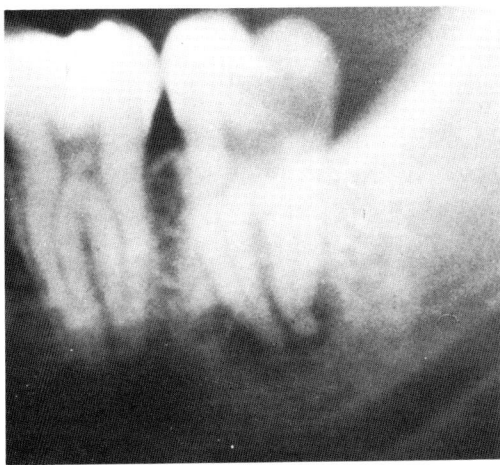

Fig. 2.4 Extensive distal caries of a partially erupted ⌐8 which has extended as far as the pulp. There is an ill defined area of bone rarefaction at the apex which is typical of an alveolar abscess.

If the root of an erupted tooth becomes exposed in the mouth due to periodontal disease or for any other reason, it is much more vulnerable to carious attack than the enamel covered crown (Fig. 2.5). Cervical caries can be detected clinically at an early stage if it begins on the buccal or lingual aspect of the tooth, but interproximal cervical caries may appear radiologically before there is any clinical abnormality.

Caries can develop at the edges of restorations and will sometimes be apparent radiographically before there is any clinical abnormality (Fig. 2.6).

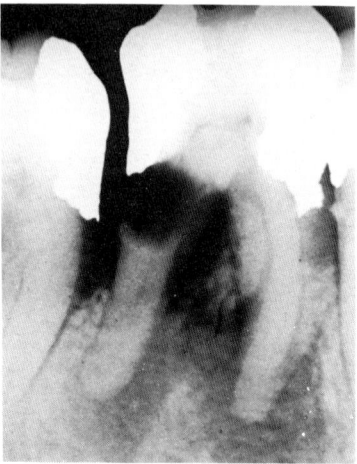

Fig. 2.5   Extensive caries of the exposed distal root of 6̄| with peri-apical bone rarefaction typical of an alveolar abscess.

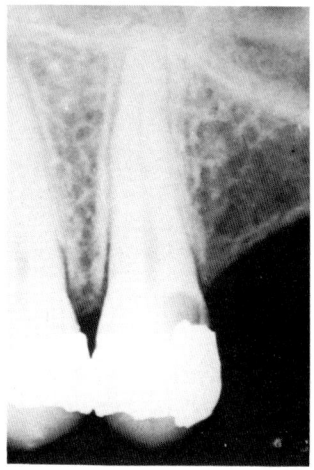

Fig. 2.6   Distal caries at the edge of an amalgam restoration of |5.

Radiation caries is the term given to the increased incidence of caries which follows therapeutic radiation to the maxillofacial region, and the development of extensive cervical caries is particularly striking (Fig. 2.7A, B). It is probably due to a combination of poor oral hygiene and reduced salivary flow and not to any alteration in the structure of the teeth themselves.

Defective calcification of enamel or dentine (e.g. amelogenesis imperfecta, dentinogenesis imperfecta) is always associated with an increased incidence of dental caries.

Bacterial invasion of the pulp (pulpitis) and pulp death produce no specific radiological change, as inflamed or dead pulp has the same radiological appearance as living pulp.

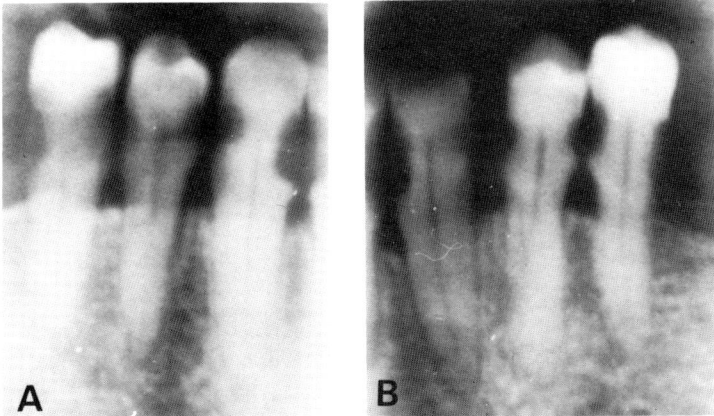

Fig. 2.7 A, B Extensive post radiation cervical caries of $\overline{543|}$ and $\overline{|345}$. There is radio-opaque calculus around the cervical margins of most teeth.

PERI-APICAL INFECTION

Peri-apical infection is usually a sequel to dental caries or trauma. It is invariably preceded by pulp death which produces no radiological abnormality, as the radiodensity of dead pulp is the same as the radiodensity of living pulp, but the cause of pulp death such as caries or injury is often apparent radiologically.

An acute alveolar abscess produces no radiological change in the alveolar bone in its early stages, and in this respect it is similar to acute osteomyelitis. There may be slight thickening of the periodontal membrane of the affected tooth due to inflammatory oedema, but this is rarely obvious. After the infection has been present for 7–10 days, a small defect becomes apparent in the lamina dura over the root apex and a small area of rarefaction soon develops in the peri-apical alveolar bone. (Fig. 2.4).

A chronic alveolar abscess may follow an acute abscess, or may begin as a low grade infection. The radiological abnormalities do not appear until the infection has been present for at least seven days and are similar to those of an acute abscess. The defect in the lamina dura and the peri-apical rarefaction soon develop into a small, irregular radiolucency adjacent to the root apex (Fig. 2.8).

A peri-apical granuloma sometimes develops as a result of a long-standing chronic peri-apical infection and appears radiologically as a well defined radiolucent area at the root apex, which may have a cortical

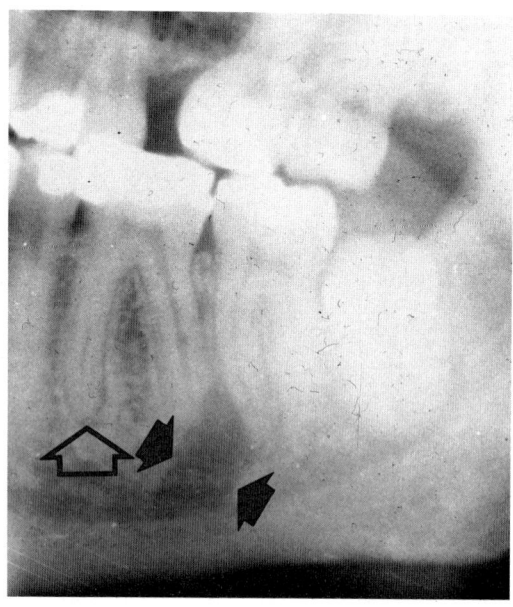

Fig. 2.8   There is a defect in the lamina dura over the apex of the mesial root of ⌐6̄
(open arrow) indicating early infection. There is a poorly defined radiolucent area at
the apex of the distal root of the same tooth which is typical of an alveolar abscess
(solid arrows).

margin (Fig. 2.9). Histologically, a granuloma consists of granulation
tissue and chronic inflammatory cells.

An apical dental cyst, the commonest cyst of the maxillofacial
region, develops when an apical granuloma undergoes central necrosis
and liquefaction. There are no radiological criteria which can be relied
upon to distinguish between a granuloma and a cyst, but if the diameter
of a peri-apical radiolucency exceeds 1 cm, or if it has a corticated
margin, it is more likely to be a cyst than a granuloma.

DENTAL RESTORATIONS[1]

Metallic restorations of silver amalgam or gold alloy are completely
radio-opaque (Fig. 1.1)

Composite resins and glass ionomer cements were formerly radiolucent,
but modern materials have radio-opaque barium added to render them
radio-opaque (Fig. 2.10).

Acrylic and silicate cements are still occasionally used to restore
anterior teeth and are completely radiolucent (Figs 2.11, 2.12).

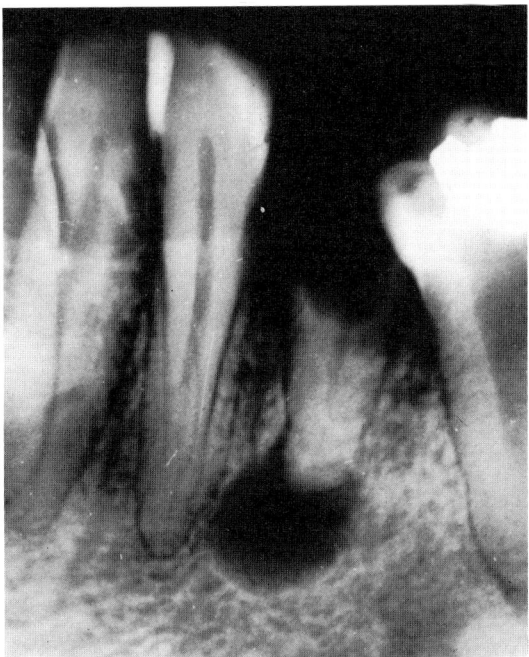

Fig. 2.9   Complete destruction of the crown of ⌐4 due to advanced caries. There is a well-defined radiolucent area at the root apex which has the appearance of a granuloma.

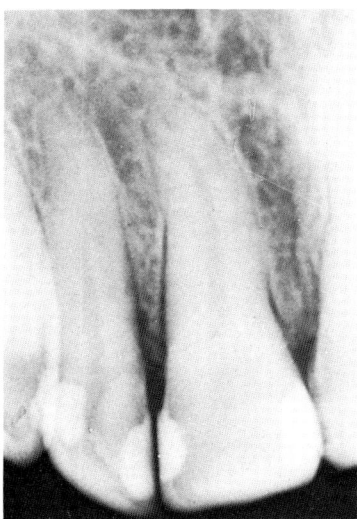

Fig. 2.10   Mesial and distal restorations of radio-opaque glass ionomer cements with radio-opaque calcium hydroxide linings in 2⌋ and 1⌋.

Cavity lining and temporary filling materials containing zinc oxide are densely radio-opaque (Figs 2.11, 2.12). *Root-capping* materials containing calcium hydroxide are also radio-opaque, but can resorb or wash out with the formation of a radiolucent area between the main filling material and the natural tooth substance.

Root-filling materials are almost invariably radio-opaque, due to the presence of zinc oxide or calcium hydroxide. Retrograde root fillings of amalgam are densely radio-opaque (Fig. 2.12).

Jacket crowns are usually made of porcelain and are slightly radio-opaque, but acrylic is still occasionally used and is completely radiolucent. Zinc phosphate cement is often used to attach the crown to the tooth and is so densely radio-opaque that a thin layer is clearly visible (Fig. 2.13).

Post crowns are always based on a densely radio-opaque metallic post, but the crown itself will consist of a more radiolucent material such as porcelain (Fig. 2.14).

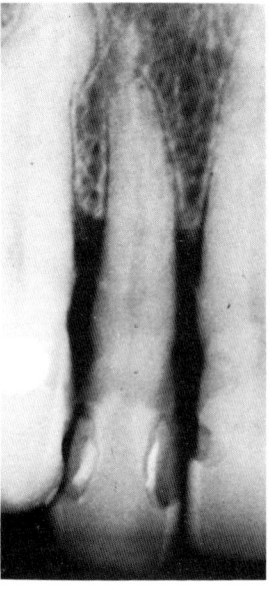

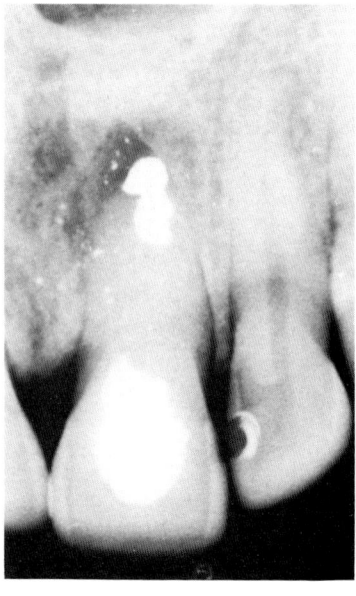

Fig. 2.11 Mesial and distal restorations in 2⌋ consisting of radiolucent silicate cement with radio-opaque linings of zinc oxide cement. There is marked reduction in the height of the alveolar crests due to advanced periodontal disease.

Fig. 2.12 Retrograde amalgam root filling of ⌊1 with a few fragments of amalgam in the alveolar bone. There is a radiolucent silicate restoration with radio-opaque zinc oxide lining mesially in ⌊2.

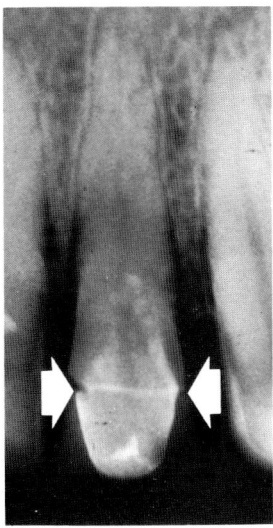

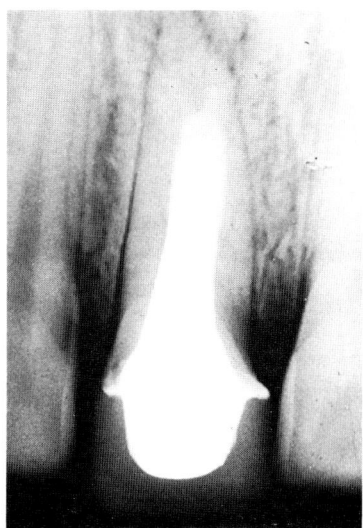

Fig. 2.13   Radiolucent acrylic jacket crown on ⌊2. The radio-opaque zinc phosphate cement is clearly visible above (arrows).

Fig. 2.14   Post crown restoration of ⌊1. The metal of the post and base is densely radio-opaque and the porcelain crown is very faintly radio-opaque.

REFERENCES

1. Abou-Tabi F F, Tidy D C, Combe E C 1979 Radio opacity of composite restorative materials. British Dental Journal 147: 187–188

3

Periodontal disease

INFLAMMATORY AND LOCAL PERIODONTAL DISEASE

The earliest radiological sign of inflammatory periodontal disease is a defect in the lamina dura of the alveolar crest between the teeth and it shows best on the intra-oral non screen film (Fig. 3.1).

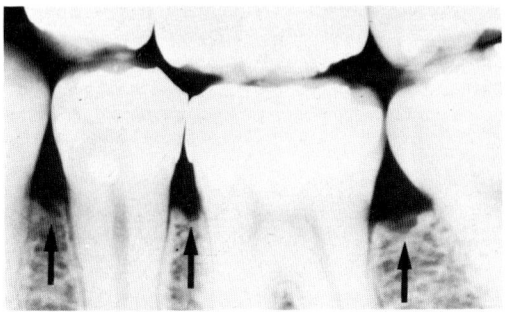

Fig. 3.1 Small defects in the alveolar crests between ⌐4, ⌐5, ⌐6 and ⌐7 indicating early periodontal disease (arrowed).

In **periodontitis simplex** bone loss proceeds at the same rate around a group of teeth with gradual lowering of the level of the alveolar crest (Fig. 3.2).

In **periodontitis complex** bone loss progresses more irregularly, with the development of periodontal pockets of varying depths (Figs 3.3, 3.4). The pockets appear as widening of the periodontal membrane and can extend as far as the root apex. They contain necrotic tissue and food debris.

Local abnormalities, such as overhanging fillings (Fig. 3.5) and abnormally erupted teeth (Fig. 3.6) predispose to pocket formation. Calculus plays an important role in the aetiology of periodontal disease, especially periodontitis simplex, and is commonly deposited around the necks of lower incisors and upper molars (Fig. 3.7).

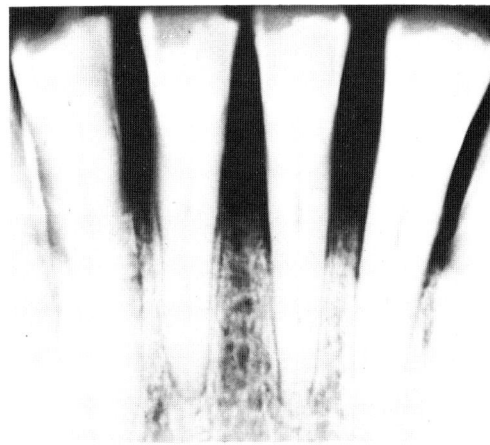

Fig. 3.2 Active periodontitis simplex with considerable loss of the alveolar bone around the lower incisor teeth.

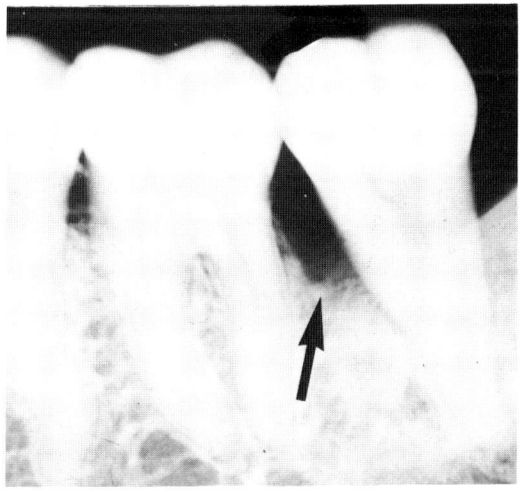

Fig. 3.3 Active periodontitis complex with a deep pocket between ⌐7 and ⌐8 (arrowed).

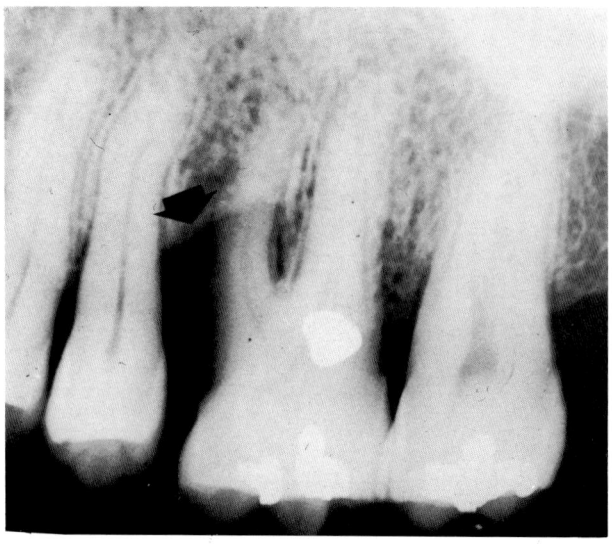

Fig. 3.4   Active periodontitis complex with deep pocketing around the upper left premolar and molar teeth. The bone loss between ⌊5 and ⌊6 is particularly severe (arrowed).

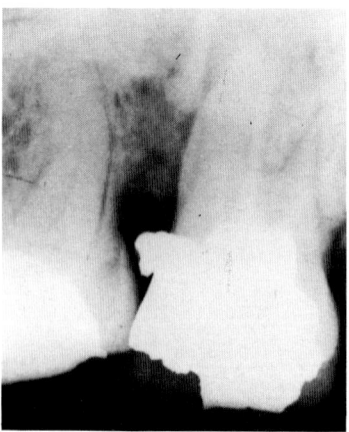

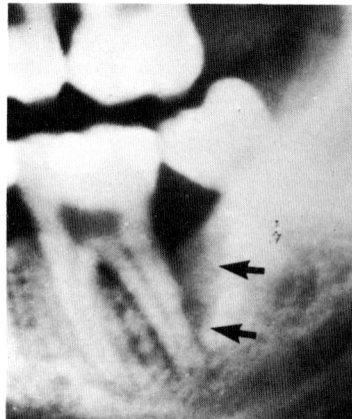

Fig. 3.5   Deep pocket between ⌊6 and ⌊7 due to an over hanging mesio-occlusal amalgam restoration.

Fig. 3.6   Deep pocket distal to ⌐7 due to a partially erupted ⌐8 (arrowed).

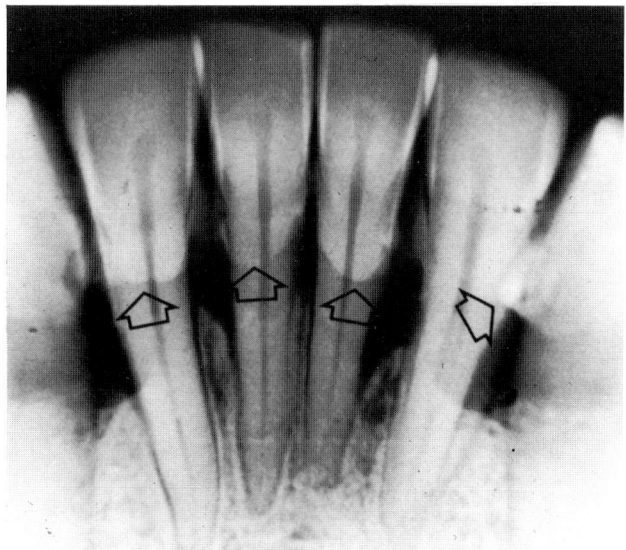

Fig. 3.7 Extensive calculus around the lower incisor teeth (arrowed) with severe bone loss.

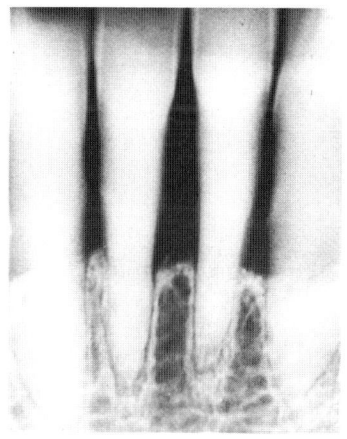

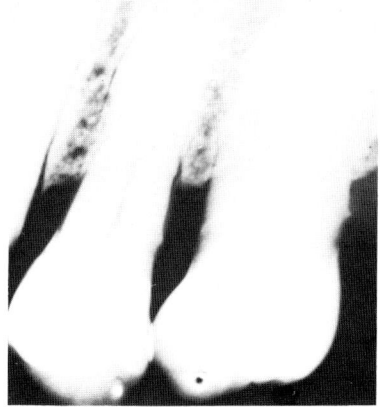

Fig. 3.8 Arrested periodontitis simplex around the lower incisor teeth with the formation of new corticated alveolar crests at lower levels.

Fig. 3.9 Arrested periodontitis complex in the left upper quadrant with the formation of new corticated alveolar crests between ⌊4, ⌊5 and ⌊6.

The progress of the disease may be arrested at any stage, when the lamina dura of the alveolar crest will regenerate, but the original height of the alveolar bone is never regained (Figs 3.8, 3.9).

A **periodontal abscess** usually develops in a deep periodontal pocket, although it is sometimes a sequel to local trauma from a toothbrush bristle, fish bone or other foreign body. Radiologically there is bone destruction around the affected tooth which can extend rapidly to the apex of the root and there is often surrounding bone rarefaction (Fig. 3.10).

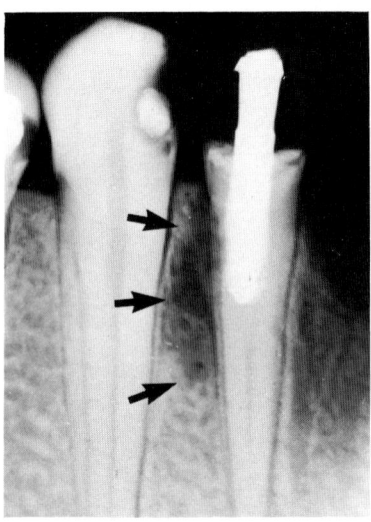

Fig. 3.10   Periodontal abscess mesial to ⌐4̄. There is partial destruction of the alveolar crest with an ill defined area of bone rarefaction below it (arrowed). The abscess developed in a periodontal pocket caused by a poorly fitting acrylic post crown.

Acute periodontitis can result from a periodontal abscess, an alveolar abscess or recurrent trauma. The diagnosis is essentially clinical, but there is usually slight thickening of the periodontal membrane which shows best on an intra-oral peri-apical film.

In **periodontosis** (or atrophic periodontitis) deep pockets develop in the absence of calculus or clinical inflammation and usually appear first in the upper anterior region. Apart from the absence of calculus and the position of the pockets, the radiological abnormalities are similar to those of periodontitis complex.

Malignant infiltration from a sarcoma or carcinoma is a rare cause of radiological widening of the periodontal membrane.

SYSTEMIC DISEASE

The incidence of inflammatory periodontal disease is higher in *diabetes mellitus* and *pregnancy*.

Scleroderma (progressive systemic sclerosis, acrosclerosis) can result in widespread thickening of the periodontal membranes.

Osteopetrosis (Albers-Schönberg disease; marble bone disease) and *infantile hypoparathyroidism* may cause generalised thickening of the lamina dura and *hyperparathyroidism* often results in rapid resorption of the lamina dura.

Hand-Schüller-Christian disease (Ch. 7) may produce extensive destruction of alveolar bone and can resemble advanced periodontal disease radiologically. The diagnosis depends upon biopsy.

4

Odontomes and developmental abnormalities of teeth

ODONTOMES

An odontome is an abnormal growth of calcified dental tissue, which behaves like a *hamartoma* rather than a neoplasm and stops growing when the individual stops growing.

Composite odontomes contain more than one dental tissue and usually present during adolescence, as they delay or prevent the eruption of permanent teeth. Simple odontomes which contain only one dental tissue are rarer than composite odontomes and are usually asymptomatic.

A complex composite odontome is a mass of enamel, dentine and cementum which shows as a dense radio opacity with an irregular but clearly defined margin (Fig. 4.1). Sometimes there are small radiolucencies within this radio-opaque mass due to small cysts. This lesion usually occurs in the molar regions, but can occur anywhere in the dental arch.

A compound composite odontome is a mass of small 'denticles', most of which contain enamel, dentine and cementum (Fig. 4.2). It is

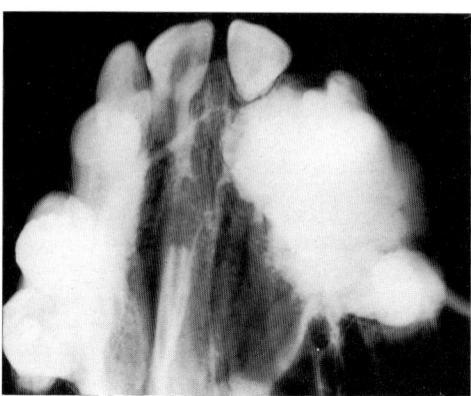

Fig. 4.1 Complex composite odontome in the upper premolar and molar regions which appears as a very dense radio opacity with a well defined lobulated margin.

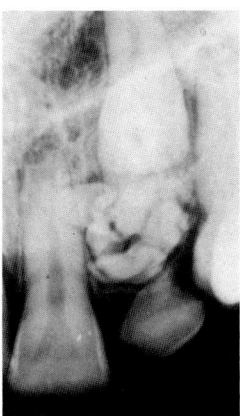

Fig. 4.2 Compound composite odontome situated between the erupted⌊B̲and its unerupted permanent successor. It appears as a mass of 'denticles' or small deformed teeth.

more common anteriorly and posteriorly. Multiple compound composite odontomes have been described in association with Gardner's syndrome.

An enameloma (or enamel pearl) is a small nodule of enamel which occasionally forms at the neck of a tooth (Fig. 2.2).

Dentinomas are extremely rare, and there is some doubt about their existence as a pathological entity. They have the radiological appearance of a complex composite odontome and tend to occur posteriorly.

A cementoma is usually classified as a fibro-osseous lesion and not as an odontome and is described in Chapter 7.

Gemination (geminated composite odontome, fusion) can occur anywhere in the dental arch, but is more common anteriorly (Fig. 4.3). It is usually the crowns of the affected teeth which are fused together.

Dens invaginatus (dilated composite odontome, dens in dente) results from invagination of the enamel into the dentine during development, and produces an enamel-lined cavity within the fully formed tooth (Fig. 4.4). The cavity communicates with the oral cavity and is usually the site of rapidly developing caries. The affected tooth, which is almost invariably an upper lateral incisor, is widened (dilated) and the radio-opaque enamel which covers the crown can be seen extending into the dentine.

ABNORMALLY SHAPED TEETH

Development anomalies of one or two teeth are common and are rarely associated with more widespread abnormalities. The most common is

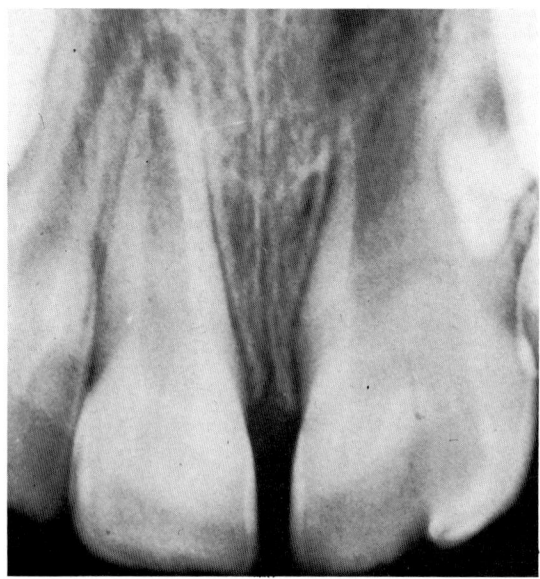

Fig. 4.3   Gemination of 1 and 2.

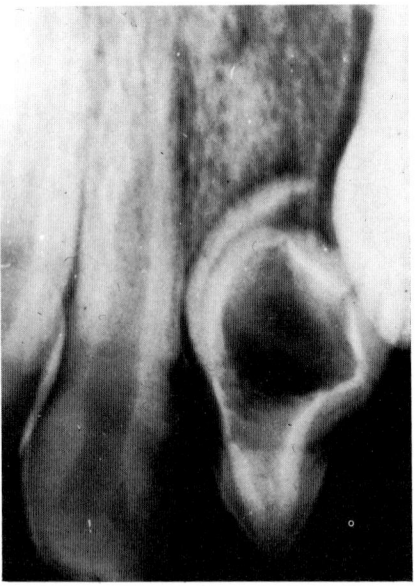

Fig. 4.4   Dens invaginatus of 2. The tooth is dilated and contains an enamel lined cavity which communicates with the oral cavity.

the peg shaped upper lateral incisor, which is obvious on clinical examination.

Taurodont teeth were common in Neanderthal man and appear occasionally in modern man. The roots of the molar teeth are fused together for most of their lengths.

The term *megadontia* is sometimes applied to teeth which are unusually large and the term *microdontia* to teeth which are abnormally small.

Congenital syphylis results in abnormalities of the crowns of the developing permanent teeth. The upper incisors have notches in their incisal edges when they erupt six years later (Hutchinson's teeth) and the crowns of the developing first molars are small, with multiple irregular cusps (Moon's molars) when they erupt at the same time.

The Ellis–van Creveld syndrome and other ectodermal dysplasias are often associated with widespread dental abnormalities — usually small teeth with pointed crowns (microdontia) and partial anodontia.

Turner's syndrome (XO syndrome) and *Down's syndrome* (trisomy 21–22) may be associated with peg-shaped upper lateral incisors and small teeth.

Dilaceration of the root of a permanent tooth may result from trauma during development but usually occurs spontaneously. It is usually seen in the upper anterior region where the angulation of the crown on the root produces a characteristic radiological appearance (Fig. 4.5).

Deformed roots in the permanent dentition may be a sequel to

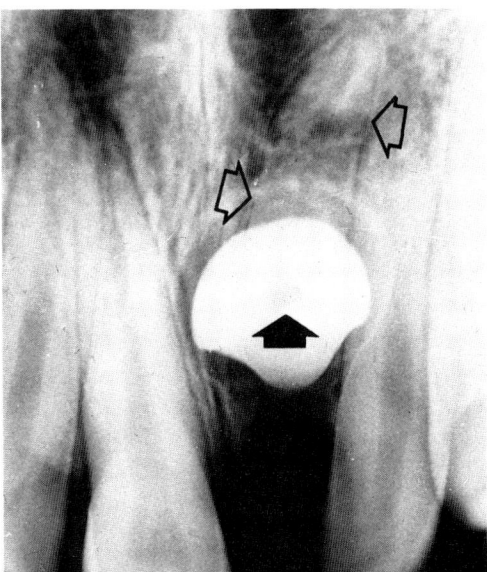

Fig. 4.5 Dilaceration of the root of ⌞⌞. The root (open arrows) is normal in position, but the crown is angled posteriorly so that the root canal (solid arrow) appears as a small, round radiolucency surrounded by dentine and enamel.

hypoparathyroidism in infancy and are also a feature of *cleidocranial dysostosis*.

Therapeutic radiation in childhood may arrest the normal development of permanent teeth and cause them to have small crowns and short, pointed roots.

SUPERNUMARY AND SUPPLEMENTAL TEETH

Supernumary teeth are extra teeth which do not resemble any normal tooth. They are usually multiple and are most common in the pre-maxillary region, where their presence usually delays the eruption of the permanent incisors (Fig. 4.6).

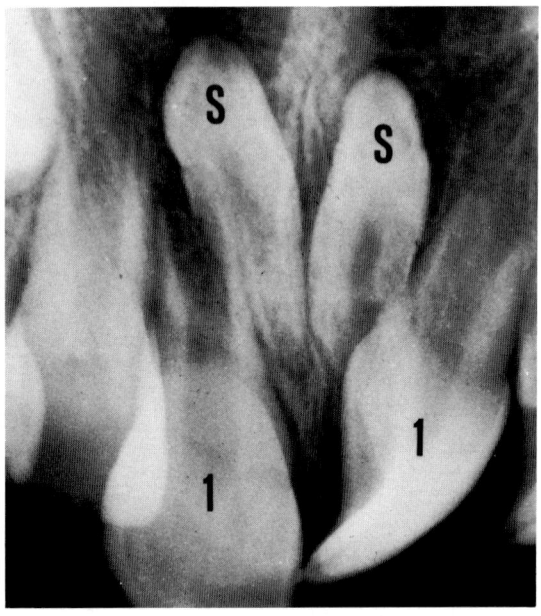

Fig. 4.6 Two inverted supernumary teeth (marked S) are situated between the roots of 1| and |1 (marked 1) and have resulted in rotation of |1.

Supplemental teeth are normally formed extra teeth and they can occur anywhere in the dental arches (Fig. 4.7).

Supernumary and supplemental teeth are a feature of cleidocranial dysostosis and have been reported in Gardner's syndrome.

Pre-deciduous teeth in the newborn are rare, as are *post-permanent teeth* in adults.

ANODONTIA AND PARTIAL ANODONTIA

It is not uncommon for the uppper lateral incisor or lower third molar (Fig. 4.8) to be absent in otherwise normal individuals.

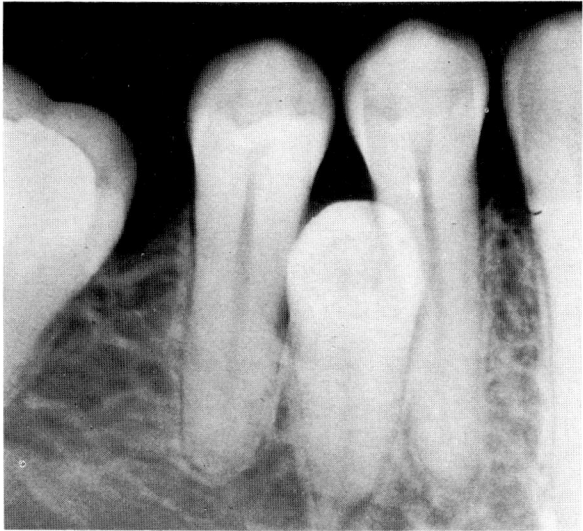

Fig. 4.7   Impacted supplemental premolar between $\overline{5|}$ and $\overline{4|}$.

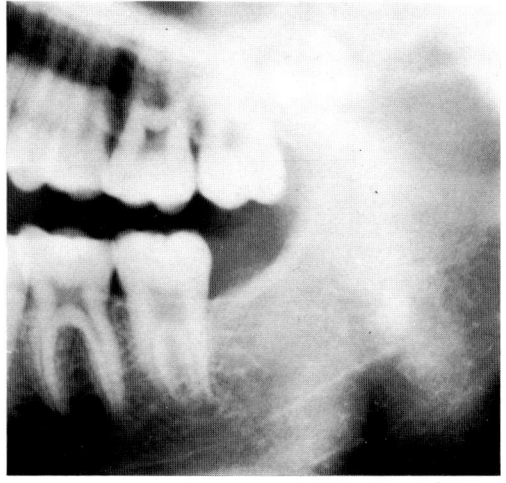

Fig. 4.8   Congenital absence of $\overline{|8}$.

Partial anodontia (absence of many teeth) and *complete anodontia* (total absence of teeth) occur rarely and there is often a family history in affected individuals (Fig. 4.9). Partial anodontia may be associated with a generalised ectodermal dysplasia such as the Ellis–van Creveld syndrome.

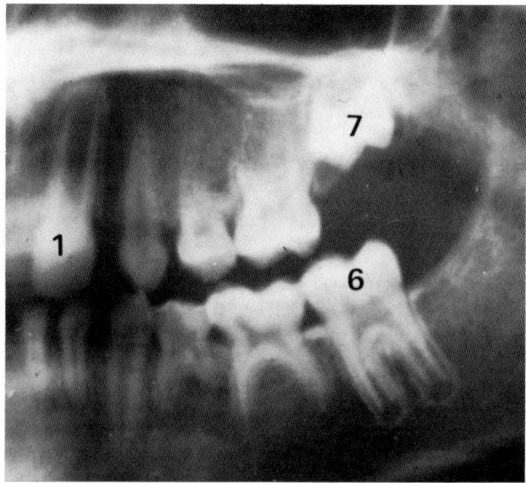

Fig. 4.9   Partial anodontia in a child aged 10 years. There are only three permanent teeth on the left side and they have been numbered. Most of the deciduous teeth are still present.

Therapeutic radiation in early childhood can result in complete failure of odontogenesis in the irradiated area and is a very rare cause of partial anodontia.

Infective *osteomyelitis in infancy* is a rare cause of partial anodontia and is more likely to affect the maxilla than the mandible.

DEFECTIVE CALCIFICATION

Dentinogenesis imperfecta (hereditary brown opalescent dentine) is a rare condition inherited as an autosomal dominant, which is sometimes associated with osteogenesis imperfecta.[1] The deciduous and permanent teeth have short crowns and roots with small pulp chambers and narrow root canals (Fig. 4.10A). The enamel is normal when the teeth erupt, but soon flakes off due to inadequate support from the underlying poorly calcified dentine (Fig. 4.10B). The teeth become rapidly carious and peri-apical infection is common.

Amelogenesis Imperfecta (hereditary enamel hypoplasia) is a rare condition, which is inherited as an autosomal dominant. The enamel is normally calcified, but is extremely thin, and this results in the crowns having a rectangular or square appearance, instead of the usual bulbous shape (Fig. 4.11). The incidence of caries is higher than in teeth with normal enamel.

Idiopathic enamel hypocalcification is another rare condition of unknown aetiology which occurs sporadically. The enamel is normal in

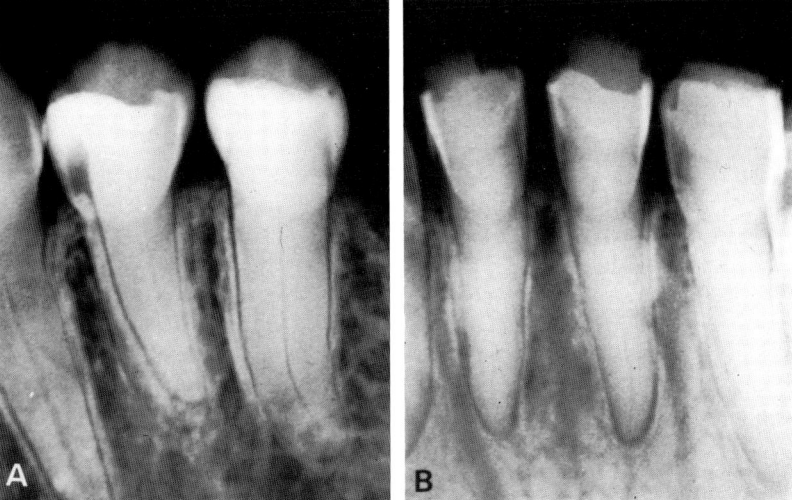

Fig. 4.10 A, B Dentinogenesis imperfecta. The teeth have short crowns and roots with small pulp chambers and narrow root canals. The enamel appears normal on recently erupted teeth (**A**), but soon flakes off the incisal edges and occlusal surfaces (**B**).

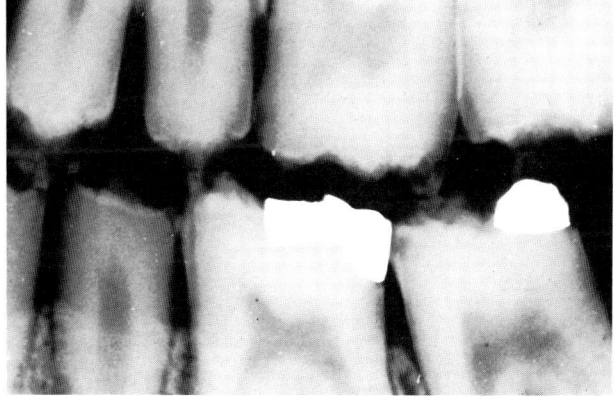

Fig. 4.11 Amelogenesis imperfecta. The enamel is normally calcified but extremely thin and this gives the crowns a rectangular or square appearance.

thickness, but is inadequately calcified. The enamel soon wears away and caries progresses rapidly.

Dentinal dysplasia (rootless teeth) is a very rare developmental anomaly which affects both dentitions. The main abnormality is that the roots are shortened and deformed, those of the anterior teeth being tapered and those of the posterior teeth being bulbous. The pulp chambers and root canals are usually absent and peri-apical bone rarefaction and alveolar abscesses are common, even in the absence of caries. Clinically the teeth appear normal, but they become loose soon after eruption and are lost early.

Shell teeth is an extremely rare abnormality of unknown aetiology. The dentine is so thin that the teeth appear to consist almost entirely of enamel.

In the *Morquio-Brailsford syndrome* the enamel is thin, poorly calcified and tends to flake away from the underlying dentine.

Local enamel defects (enamel pits) may result from severe childhood fevers, such as measles and gastroenteritis, and are due to a temporary failure of enamel formation in the developing teeth.

Peri-apical dental infection of deciduous teeth can result in defects in the thickness and calcification of the enamel of their permanent successors.

Severe rickets in infancy may result in enamel hypocalcification and severe *scurvy* can result in thin, hypocalcified dentine and in hypoplastic enamel due to inadequate development of the collagen matrix. *Hypophosphatasia*, like severe rickets, results in hypocalcification of enamel and also causes premature loss of the deciduous teeth, due to defective cementum (Fig. 4.12A, B).

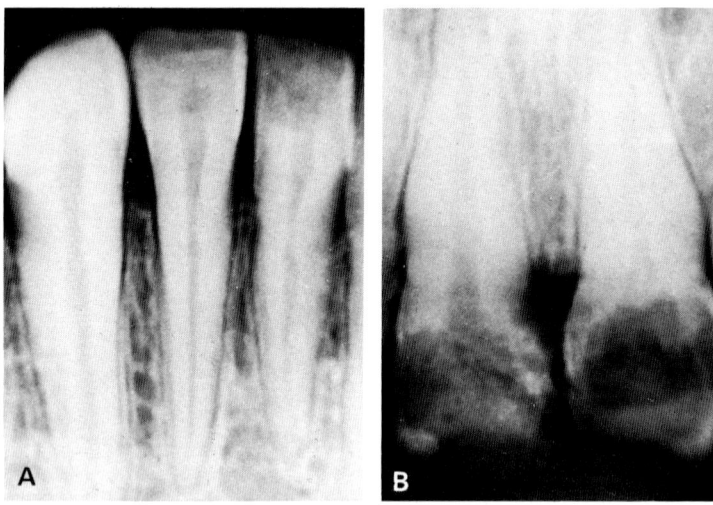

Fig. 4.12 Hypophosphatasia. **A**. The hypocalcified enamel has worn away from the incisal edges of $\overline{2|}$ and $\overline{1|}$ but the enamel of the more recently erupted $\overline{3|}$ is still intact. **B**. Extensive destruction of the crowns of $\underline{1|1}$ due to a combination of wear and caries.

Hypoparathyroidism in infants and young children may cause hypoplastic enamel in the developing permanent teeth.

Fluorosis due to prolonged ingestion of water with a fluoride concentration exceeding one part per million may result in pitting and discolouration of enamel.

REFERENCES

Schwartz S, Tsipouras P 1984 Oral findings in osteogenesis imperfecta. Oral Surgery, Oral Medicine, Oral Pathology 57: 161–167

5

Benign cysts and tumours

GENERAL CONSIDERATIONS

Benign cysts of the jaws differ pathologically from benign cysts occurring in other bones, as they tend to be of dental origin. They are common lesions which usually present when they rupture into the oral cavity and become infected, with the result that the radiological features of infection are often superimposed on the radiological features of a simple cyst. In particular, the cortical margin round the cyst is often incomplete due to infection.

Benign cysts tend to displace the roots of adjacent teeth without resorbing them, although root resorption can occur. Cysts can become very large before they present clinically; for instance, mandibular cysts may extend from the condylar neck to the incisor region and maxillary cysts can expand into the maxillary sinus. Large cysts can appear multilocular on radiographs, but are always unilocular at operation.

Benign tumours are less common than cysts and, although their radiological features are broadly similar, they are more likely to be multilocular and are more likely to displace and resorb teeth than cysts.

The role of radiology in the management of benign cysts and tumours is to determine the extent of the lesion, so that biopsy or surgical excision can be planned. Although the radiological abnormalities should make it possible to suggest the main diagnostic possibilities, it is rarely possible to make a precise pathological diagnosis on the radiological evidence alone. As in other bones, this depends on a combination of the clinical, radiological and histological findings, together with biochemical and immunological tests in some cases.

There is little doubt that *CT scanning* can define the bony extent of a benign cyst or tumour with more accuracy than conventional radiography and there is no doubt that it shows soft tissue extension in a way that is quite impossible with conventional radiography.

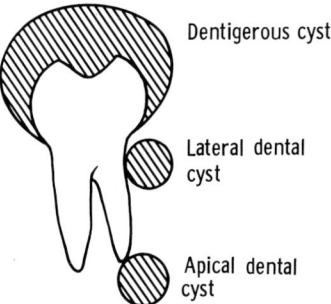

Dentigerous cyst

Lateral dental cyst

Apical dental cyst

Fig. 5.1 Diagram of the sites of a dentigerous cyst, lateral dental cyst and apical dental cyst.

DENTAL CYST

An apical dental cyst (apical periodontal cyst) is the most common cyst of the jaws and accounts for almost half of all radiolucent jaw lesions. It develops at the root apex of a non-vital permanent tooth (Fig. 5.1) and can present at any age above twenty years (Fig. 5.2). The pulp may be necrotic due to infection or trauma, or the tooth may have been root-treated.

The cyst develops as a result of necrosis within a granuloma, so the radiological features of an apical granuloma merge with those of a small cyst. If the diameter of a corticated radiolucent area at the apex of a

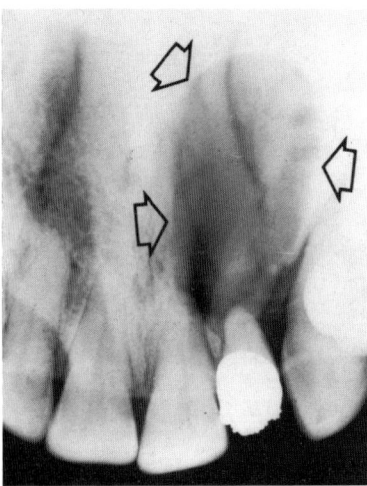

Fig. 5.2 Apical dental cyst arising from a heavily filled non-vital ⌞2 which has displaced the root apex anteriorly. The cortical margin of the cyst has been destroyed by infection.

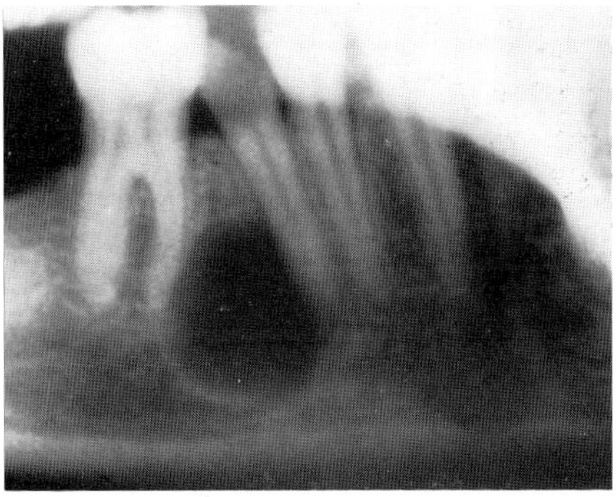

Fig. 5.3 Apical dental cyst arising from a carious non-vital 5⏌ which has displaced the root anteriorly. The cortical margin is largely intact.

tooth exceeds 1cm it is probably a cyst. Large cysts can expand the cortical outline of the maxilla or mandible and maxillary cysts may expand into the maxillary sinus.

The bony margin is corticated and continuous unless the cyst has become infected, or a pathological fracture has occurred. Some cysts appear multilocular radiologically, but they are always unilocular at operation. The roots of adjacent teeth are often displaced (Fig. 5.3) and are very occasionally eroded (Fig. 5.4).

The lining consists of thick, stratified, squamous epithelium which rarely shows evidence of keratinisation.

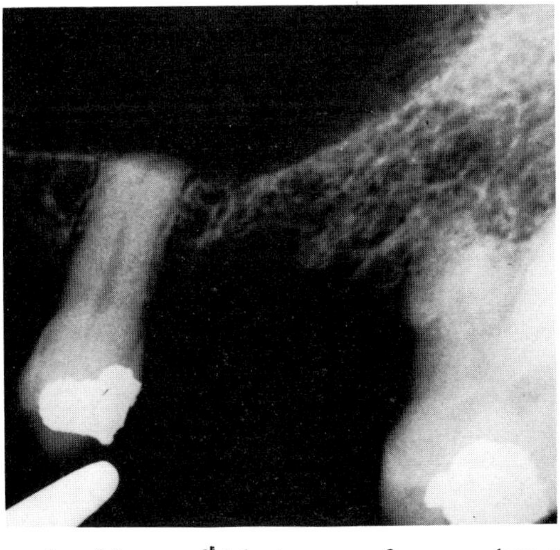

Fig. 5.4 Resorption of the root of ⎣4 due to pressure from a very large apical dental cyst arising from a non-vital ⎣2.

A **lateral dental cyst** (lateral periodontal cyst) is a rare lesion which develops lateral to the root of a dead or living tooth (Fig. 5.1). It has the same radiological features as an apical dental cyst, except that it is situated alongside a tooth and not at its apex.

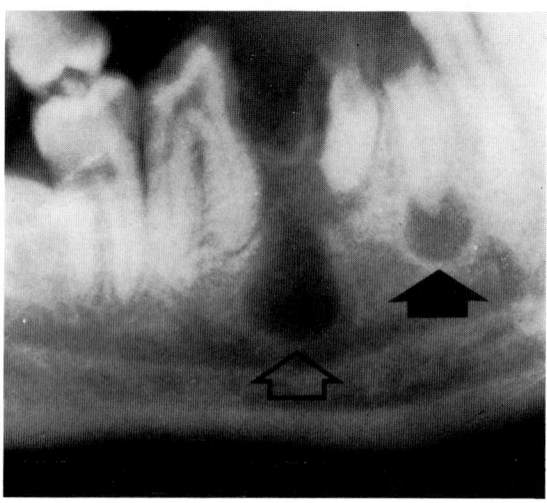

Fig. 5.5   The large radiolucent area with no cortical margin (open arrow) is a small residual dental cyst, the cortical margin having been destroyed by infection. The smaller round radiolucent area with the corticated margin (solid arrow) is typical of an apical granuloma.

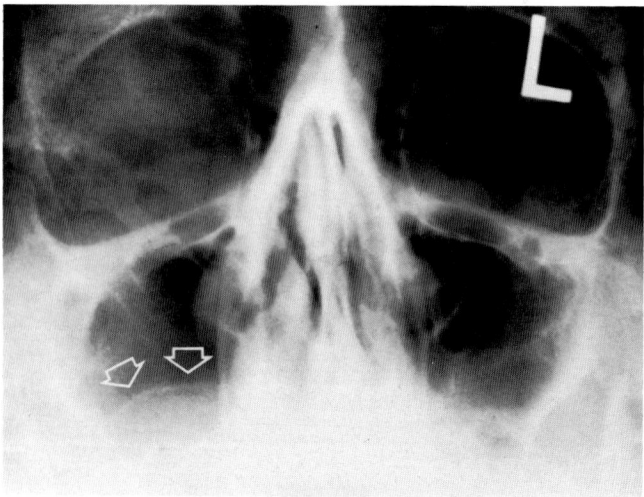

Fig. 5.6   Large residual dental cyst expanding into the right maxillary sinus. The radio-opaque line at the upper margin of the soft tissue shadow (arrows) indicates that the lesion has originated outside the maxillary sinus and expanded into it.

A **residual dental cyst** (residual periodontal cyst) is an apical or lateral dental cyst which was left behind when the tooth from which it developed was extracted (Fig. 5.5). It is, therefore, more common in the older age groups. These cysts can become very large (Fig. 5.6) and have the same radiological features as apical dental cysts, except that they occur in edentulous areas of the jaws.

DENTIGEROUS CYST

A dentigerous cyst develops from the enamel-forming tissue (enamel organ) of a developing permanent tooth. This produces the characteristic radiological appearance of a corticated radiolucent area surrounding the crown of an unerupted tooth.

These cysts usually present during the second decade and commonly develop around the crowns of lower third molars or lower second premolars (Figs. 5.7, 5.8). The cortical outline is continuous in the absence of infection. Adjacent teeth are often displaced, but their roots are rarely resorbed. Dentigerous cysts can become very large and may

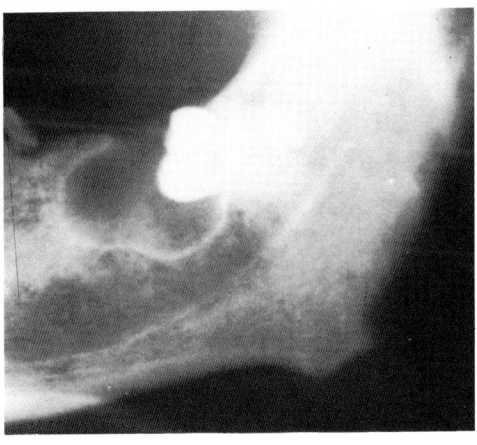

Fig. 5.7 Small dentigerous cyst around the crown of a horizontally impacted ⌐8. There is a root fragment anterior to the cyst.

expand the cortical outlines of the maxilla or mandible. Maxillary cysts occasionally expand into the maxillary sinus. Large cysts often have a multilocular appearance, but are always unilocular at operation.

The lining of an uninfected cyst consists of thin, regular, stratified, squamous epithelium, with occasional keratinisation, but if the cyst has become infected, the lining will resemble that of a dental cyst.

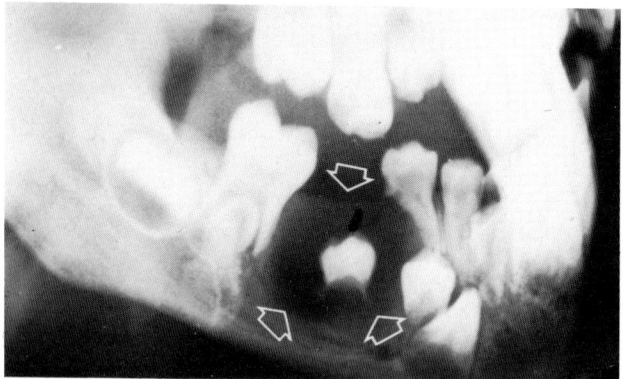

Fig. 5.8 Dentigerous cyst around the crown of an unerupted $\overline{5|}$. The radiolucent area (arrowed) lacks a cortical margin as it has been destroyed by infection.

FISSURAL CYSTS

An **incisive canal cyst** (naso-palatine cyst) arises within the incisive canal of the maxilla. The diagnosis can be made with some confidence if the diameter of the incisive canal measures more than 2 cm and should be suggested if the diameter exceeds 1.5 cm. The margin is smooth, corticated and continuous unless infection has supervened. These cysts usually present as painless, palatal swellings (Fig. 5.9).

The lining of an uninfected cyst consists largely of stratified squamous epithelium, but ciliated columnar epithelium is sometimes present.

A **globulo-maxillary cyst** is an uncommon fissural cyst which develops at the junction between the pre-maxilla and maxilla, where it appears as a corticated radiolucent area between the roots of the lateral

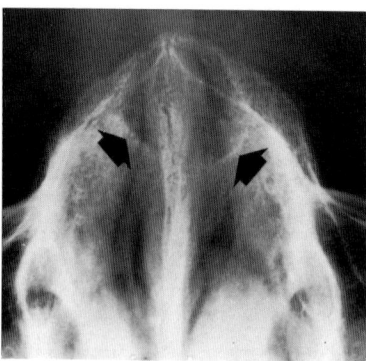

Fig. 5.9 Incisive canal cyst or naso-palatine cyst (arrowed).

incisor and the canine teeth. There may be some separation of the roots, but there is never any resorption. The cortical margin is continuous unless infection has occurred.

The lining may consist of non-keratinising stratified squamous epithelium, keratinised squamous epithelium or ciliated columnar epithelium.

Median mandibular and median palatal cysts are extremely rare fissural cysts, which appear radiologically as corticated radiolucent areas in the midline of the mandible and palate.

ODONTOGENIC KERATOCYST[1]

Odontogenic keratocysts (or primordial cysts) occur most commonly in the ramus of the mandible (Fig. 5.10) and are often associated with a missing lower third molar. However, they can arise from any tooth-bearing part of the jaws.

The diagnosis depends entirely upon the histological appearance of the lining, which consists of a thin layer of keratinised, stratified, squamous epithelium. Microscopic daughter cysts are occasionally seen

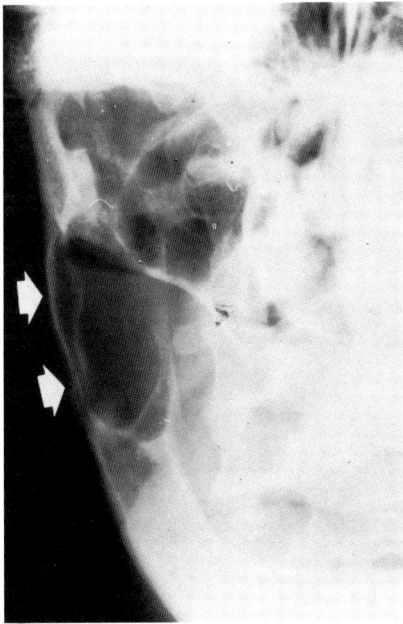

Fig. 5.10 Odontogenic keratocyst expanding the outer plate of the right ramus of the mandible (arrowed).

beyond the bony margin of the main cyst and this may account for the relatively high incidence of recurrence after simple curettage (10–20%). The cortical margin is usually smooth, but may be scalloped and is continuous unless infection has developed. Large odontogenic keratocysts will expand the maxilla or mandible and sometimes appear multilocular. They resemble a wide range of radiolucent lesions, including dental cysts and benign solid tumours.

Multiple odontogenic keratocysts are a feature of *Gorlin's syndrome.*

NON-EPITHELIAL BONE CYST[2]

The non-epithelial bone cyst (solitary bone cyst, haemorrhagic bone cyst, traumatic bone cyst, unicameral bone cyst) is almost invariably located in the body of the mandible below the premolar and molar teeth. They are usually discovered in young adults as an incidental radiological finding.

Radiologically, non-epithelial bone cysts differ from other benign cystic lesions, as they have no corticated margin and rarely cause expansion. They appear as irregular defects in the trabecular pattern of the mandible. They are invariably asymptomatic and never become infected (Fig. 5.11)

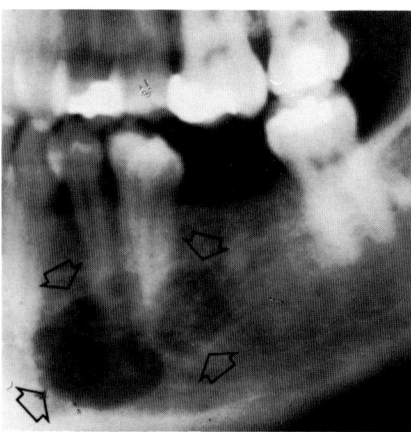

Fig. 5.11 Non-epithelial bone cyst of the mandible adjacent to the roots of the lower premolar teeth. The margin is irregular and not corticated (arrowed).

These lesions should not really be classified as cysts, as they have no epithelial lining. The pathology is uncertain and it has been suggested that they are bone infarcts, or even a normal anatomical feature. The usual management is exploration and curettage as this confirms the diagnosis. A few untreated cysts have been seen to heal spontaneously on follow-up radiographs.

BENIGN TUMOURS

The **giant cell tumour** (osteoclastoma) of the jaws, like giant cell tumours elsewhere, usually develops in adults between 20 and 40 years. Radiologically it appears as an expanding multilocular lesion with a scalloped margin. Recurrence after excision is common.

The **giant cell granuloma** is peculiar to the jaws and has the same radiological features as a giant cell tumour. However, it occurs in a younger age group (10–25 years) and, although it grows more rapidly than a giant cell tumour, it rarely recurs after removal.

The **myxoma** is a rare tumour of adults which appears radiologically as a multilocular expanding lesion. It can extend into the soft tissues and may recur after removal (Fig. 5.12).

An **osteoma** is a slow-growing benign tumour which rarely arises from the cortex of the maxilla or mandible, but which is quite common in the frontal sinuses. It appears as a radio-opaque bony outgrowth with a well-defined margin (Fig. 5.13). Large tumours tend to be pedunculated and often have a lobulated margin. Multiple osteomas are

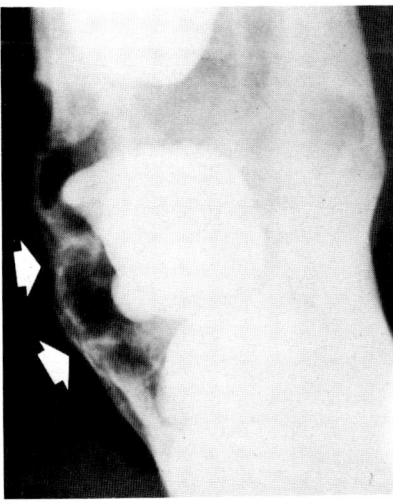

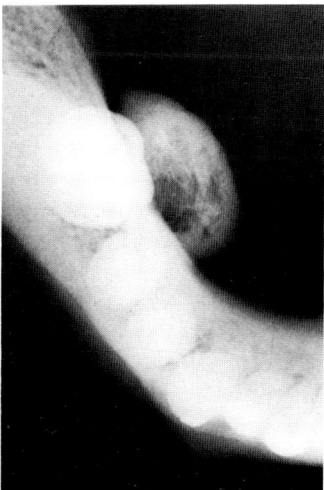

Fig. 5.12 Myxoma of the body of the mandible on an intra-oral occlusal film. The lesion has a multilocular appearance and has expanded the buccal plate (arrows).

Fig. 5.13 Benign osteoma arising from the lingual plate of the madible.

a feature of Gardner's syndrome, but can occur in the absence of any systemic abnormality.

An *osteochondroma* is an even rarer tumour, which appears as a bony outgrowth with a rather irregular cortical margin. When it occurs in the maxillofacial region it usually arises in the coronoid process of the mandible. The *chondroma* is a very rare tumour of the maxilla, which usually develops after the age of 40. It appears as an area of bone rarefaction, often containing areas of calcification and tends to erode the roots of teeth without displacing them. Complete excision is difficult and recurrence is common. Sarcomatous change can occur.

The non-odontogenic *fibroma* and odontogenic fibroma are rare bone tumours which appear as expanding radiolucent lesions with well-defined cortical margins.

Haemangioma of bone is an extremely rare tumour of children and adults, which is important as it usually results in torrential haemorrhage after dental extractions (Fig. 5.14). Radiologically it can appear as a multilocular expanding radiolucent lesion (usually in the mandible) or as an area of course and sparse trabeculae (usually in the maxilla). The pre-operative diagnosis depends upon arteriography and it is now common practice to carry out therapeutic embolisation prior to surgical removal.

Haemangioma of the soft tissues is usually a separate entity and can result in ring opacities in the soft tissues due to calcified phleboliths (see Fig. 16.3).

A *neurilemmoma* or *neurofibroma* can arise from the inferior dental nerve and will cause widening of the inferior dental canal.

There have been a few reports of other benign tumours, such as *lipomas, ganglioneuromas* and *osteoid osteomas* developing in the maxillofacial region.

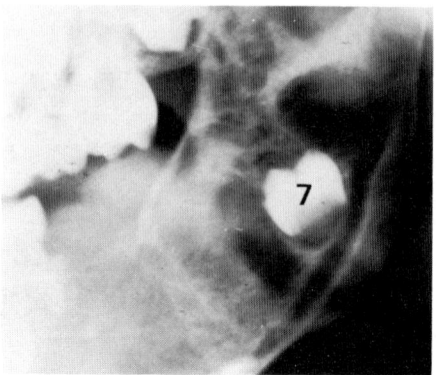

Fig. 5.14 Haemangioma of the body and ramus of the mandible in a child of 6 years. The ⌈6 had recently been extracted, as it was loose, and this had resulted in torrential haemorrhage. The developing ⌈7 (labelled) has been displayed posteriorly into the ramus by the growing tumour.

REFERENCES

1. McIvor J 1972 The radiological features of odontogenic keratocysts. British Journal of Oral Surgery 10: 116–125
2. Steidler N E, Cook R M, Reade R C 1979 Aneurysmal bone cysts of the jaws. British Journal of Oral Surgery 16: 254–261

6

Ameloblastoma and malignant tumours

AMELOBLASTOMA AND ASSOCIATED TUMOURS

Ameloblastoma (adamantinoma) is a difficult tumour to classify as its behaviour ranges from benign to locally malignant, and pulmonary metastases have been reported in a few cases.[4] It usually develops in the tooth-bearing parts of the jaws, or in the ramus of the mandible. The histological appearance of ameloblastoma is very variable and does not correlate with its behaviour. The tumour can occur at any time after the age of 12 years, but usually present in early adult life.

Radiologically the lesion begins as a radiolucent area with a corticated margin. It is usually multilocular and is probably the most common multilocular lesion in the maxillofacial region (Figs 6.1, 6.2). It frequently erodes the roots of adjacent teeth without displacing them and tends to expand the overlying cortical bone before perforating it to invade the adjacent soft tissues.[6] Maxillary lesions can extend into the maxillary sinus and invade the pterygopalatine fossa, infratemporal fossa and the base of the skull.

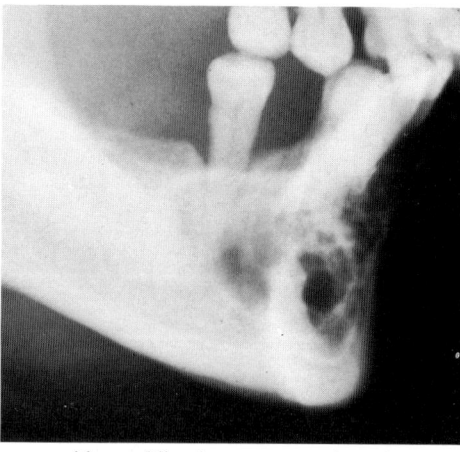

Fig. 6.1 Ameloblastoma with a multilocular appearance situated anteriorly in the mandible.

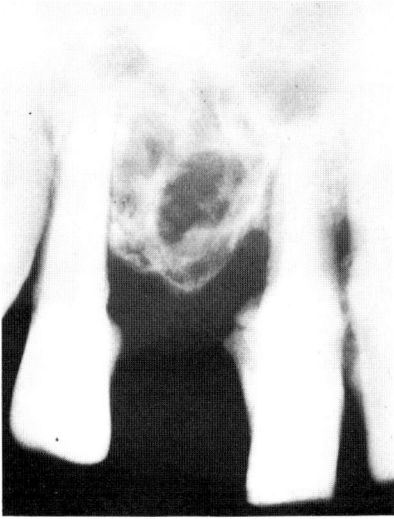

Fig. 6.2 Multilocular ameloblastoma invading the alveolar bone of the maxilla. There is advanced periodontal disease and extensive calculus formation around the standing teeth. The⌊1⌋ had recently been extracted as it had become loose.

The extent of the lesion is best shown by CT scanning (Fig. 6.3), which is of particular value in assessing large tumours prior to surgery.

Recurrence is common after local currettage and histological studies have shown that clusters of tumour cells often extend beyond the apparently intact bony margin. It is now current practice to remove a margin of macroscopically normal bone along with the tumour at the

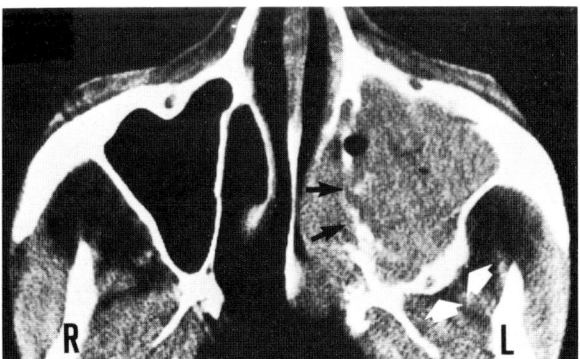

Fig. 6.3 Ameloblastoma on a transverse (or axial) CT scan viewed from below. The tumour fills the left maxillary sinus. It has expanded the posterolateral wall of the sinus (white arrows) and has destroyed part of the medial wall (black arrows) to invade the nasal cavity.

time of surgery. These tumours grow slowly and can reach an enormous size.

Ameloblastic fibroma is rarer than ameloblastoma and, although histologically distinctive, has the same pattern of clinical behaviour and the same radiological appearance as ameloblastoma.

Ameloblastic fibro-odontoma and the calcifying epithelial *odontogenic tumour of Pindborg* are very rare tumours which always contain small areas of histological calcification.[3] The calcification may be apparent radiographically and, if so, produces the characteristic picture of a radiolucent lesion containing well defined small opacities. These tumours behave like ameloblastoma and are locally invasive.

Adenomatoid odontogenic tumour (adenoblastoma) is a rare lesion which is completely benign and there is some doubt about its classification, as it may not be a true neoplasm. Radiologically it appears as a corticated radiolucent area in the tooth-bearing parts of the jaws.

Ameloblastic carcinoma and *ameloblastic sarcoma* are extremely rare malignant variants of ameloblastoma.

CARCINOMA

Carcinoma is the most common malignancy of the maxillofacial region and usually presents in the middle-aged and elderly with pain, anaesthesia and loosening of teeth. Most tumours are squamous cell carcinomas or adenocarcinomas. They usually arise from the oral mucosa and rapidly invade the underlying bone (Fig. 6.4), but occasionally develop within the mandible or maxilla, or in the lining of a simple dental cyst.[1]

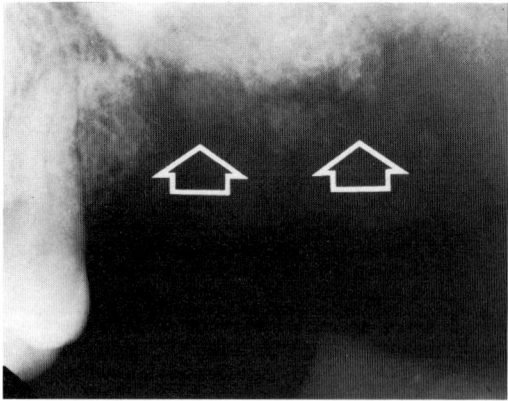

Fig. 6.4 Carcinoma of the upper alveolus. There is irregular destruction of the alveolar crest with loss of its normal cortical margin (arrowed).

Radiologically the lesion is *completely destructive* and the boundary between affected and normal bone is blurred and indistinct. Carcinoma tends to spread extensively through the trabecular bone of the maxilla and mandible and maxillary lesions frequently invade the sinus (Fig. 6.5). The tumour often erodes the roots of the teeth without displacing them and can cause widening of their periodontal membranes. Unlike benign lesions and the locally invasive ameloblastoma, carcinoma never results in bony expansion.

The treatment is radiotherapy or radical resection.

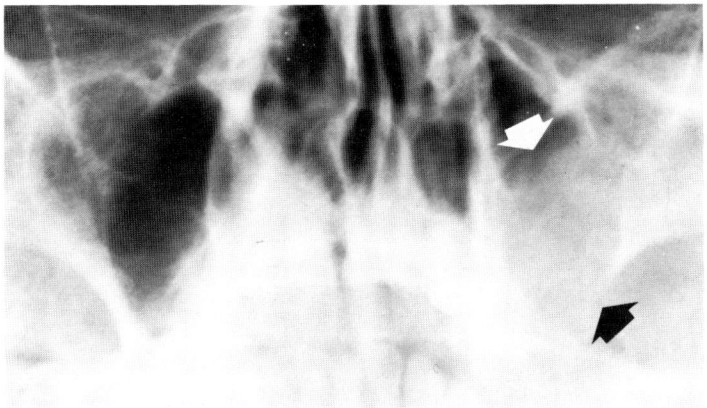

Fig. 6.5 Carcinoma of the left upper alveolus causing extensive bone destruction (black arrow) and partial opacification of the left maxillary sinus (white arrow).

SARCOMA[2]

Sarcoma is the most common malignant tumour of the jaws in young adults and usually presents between fifteen and thirty years with pain, local anaesthesia and loosening of the teeth.

Radiologically it appears as an ill-defined area of bone destruction, which is often associated with resorption of the roots of adjacent teeth and with thickening of their periodontal membranes. In a few cases, sclerosis is more marked than bone destruction and these tumours are said to have a slightly better prognosis.

However, the most striking radiological abnormality is the presence of *sub-periosteal new bone*, which may have a lamellar (onion skin) or spiculated (sun ray) appearance and which is often very extensive (Fig. 6.6A, B). CT scanning[7] will, of course, demonstrate the bony extent of the tumour and any spread into the soft tissues with more accuracy than

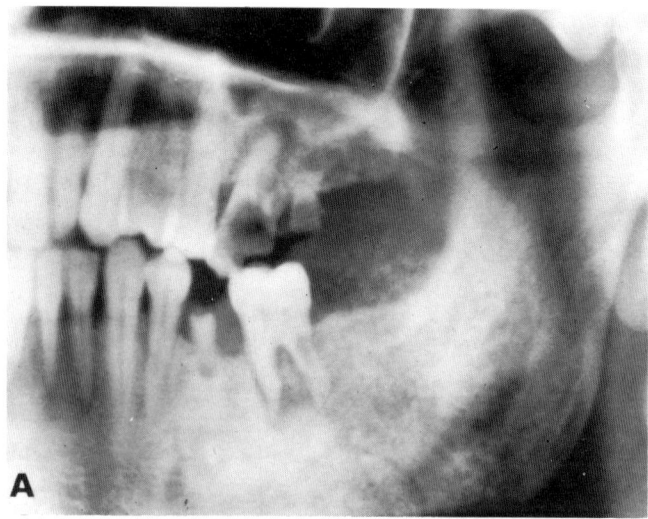

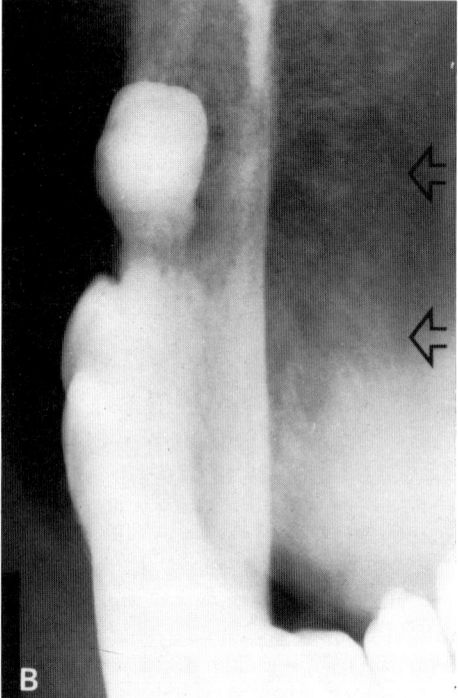

Fig. 6.6 A. Osteogenic sarcoma of the mandible with irregular bone destruction in the molar region, thickening of the periodontal membrane of $\overline{6}$ and new bone formation in the soft tissues anterior to the ramus. **B.** Occlusal view of the same case to show the spiculated (sun ray) appearance of subperiosteal new bone arising from the inner aspect of the mandible.

conventional radiography (Fig. 6.7). Histologically the tumour is always more widespread than the radiological and CT abnormalities suggest and radical excision offers the only hope of a permanent cure.

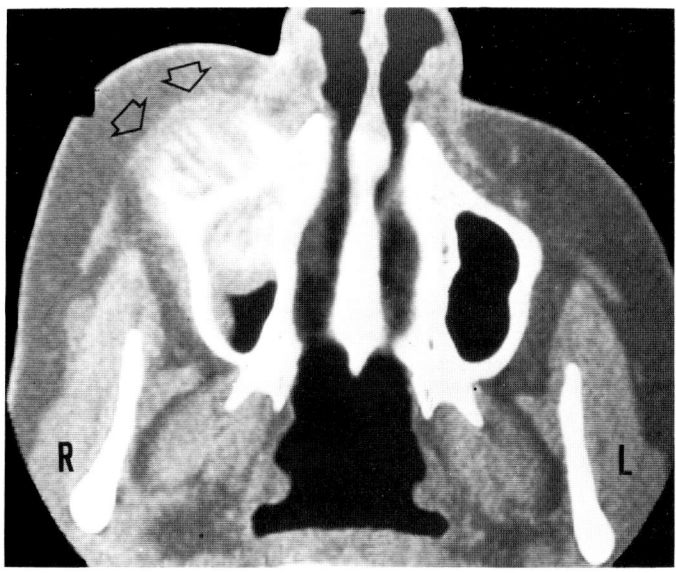

Fig. 6.7 Sarcoma of the right maxilla on a transverse (or axial) CT scan viewed from below. There is extensive new bone formation on both sides of the anterolateral wall of the sinus with 'sun ray' spiculation anteriorly. The tumour has extended into the maxillary sinus and into the soft tissues of the cheek (arrowed) beyond the new bone.

METASTATIC TUMOURS AND RARE PRIMARY TUMOURS

Metastatic carcinoma rarely affects the maxillofacial region, but when it does, the primary is usually situated in the breast, bronchus, colon or kidney. Radiologically there may be a single, ill-defined area of bone destruction, or multiple coalescing radiolucent areas scattered throughout the maxillofacial bones (Fig. 6.8). Occasionally a single metastasis lodges in the inferior dental canal and widens it.

In most cases there is radiological evidence of widespread bone metastases in these patients and it is most unusual to see lytic areas in the mandible in the absence of similar abnormalities in the skull vault. As in other bones, radiolucent metastases may become sclerotic after chemotherapy.

Multiple myeloma is unusual radiologically in that it can result in multiple radiolucencies in the mandible in the absence of similar radiolucent areas in the skull vault.

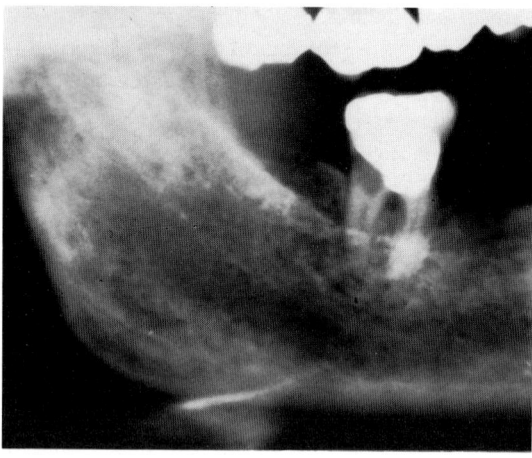

Fig. 6.8   Metastatic caricinoma of the breast. There are multiple small radiolucencies scattered throughout the ramus and body of the mandible.

Solitary plasmacytoma[5] occurs rarely in the maxilla and mandible, where it appears as a well-defined radiolucent area, often with a scalloped margin.

Burkitt's lymphoma is very common in some parts of Africa, where it affects children of all ages. Radiologically it is a purely destructive lesion in the maxilla or mandible, with patchy radiolucencies in the trabecular bone, destruction of the cortex, rapid resorption of the lamina dura and destruction of the developing teeth. It is usually accompanied by massive soft tissue swelling.

Metastatic neuroblastoma and retinoblastoma occasionally involve the maxillofacial region in children with widespread disease.

Ewing's tumour[8] and various other sarcomas have also been reported in the maxillo-facial region as primary tumours.

Malignant lymphoma[9] (e.g. lymphosarcoma, reticulum cell sarcoma etc.) can occur in the maxillofacial region, usually in patients with extensive disease elsewhere. Radiologically it is a purely destructive lesion.

REFERENCES

1. Browne R M, Gouch N G 1972 Malignant change in the epithelial lining of odontogenic cysts. Cancer 29: 1199
2. Finkelstein J B 1970 Osteosarcoma of the jaw bones. Radiological Clinics of North America 8 (3): 425–443
3. Franklin C D, Pindborg J J 1976 The calcifying epithelial odontogenic tumour: a review and analysis of 113 cases. Oral Surgery 42: 753–765
4. Jephcote C M J 1981 Ameloblastoma with pulmonary metastases. British Journal of Oral Surgery 19: 38–43
5. Loh H S 1984 A restrospective evaluation of 23 reported cases of solitary plasmacytoma of the mandible, with an additional case report. British Journal of Oral and Maxillofacial Surgery 22: 216–224

6. McIvor J 1974 The radiological features of ameloblastoma. Clinical Radiology 25: 237–242
7. Mendelsohn D B, Hertzanu Y, Glass R B J 1983 Computed tomographic findings in primary mandibular osteosarcoma. Clinical Radiology 34: 153–155
8. De Santis L A 1978 Radiographic findings of Ewing's sarcoma of the jaws. British Journal of Radiology 51: 682–687
9. Sciubba J J 1984 Oral presentations in non Hodgkin's lymphoma: a review of 31 cases. Oral Surgery, Oral Medicine, Oral Pathology 57: 272–280

7

Fibro-osseus and non-neoplastic conditions

FIBROUS DYSPLASIA

Fibrous dysplasia is more common in the maxilla than in the mandible and presents as a painless bony swelling, usually in adolescence, but sometimes earlier or later.[5] It is usually monostotic in the maxillofacial region, but can be a feature of polystotic fibrous dysplasia, or even of *Albright's syndrome*.

The earliest radiological abnormality is an expanding radiolucent lesion, which does not cross suture lines but which can deform them. Sclerotic areas soon develop within the radiolucency and these gradually enlarge and coalesce until there is dense, homogeneous opacification of the expanded bone (Fig. 7.1A), sometimes described as the 'ground glass' appearance.

Non-screen intra-oral films will sometimes show generalised thickening of the individual bone trabeculae and this appearance, which has been compared to 'orange peel', is virtually diagnostic of the disease (Fig. 7.1B).

The teeth in the affected bone are often displaced and this can result in malocclusion. The eruption of developing teeth is usually delayed or prevented.

Fibrous dysplasia is occasionally complicated by chronic infection, which adds the radiological features of patchy rarefaction and sub-periosteal new bone formation to the existing generalised expansion and sclerosis. The resulting radiological appearance can resemble a sclerotic type of osteosarcoma or sclerosing osteomyelitis.

The condition usually becomes static in early adult life, but the abnormalities which have developed do not regress. Treatment is aimed at reducing the facial deformity by surgical reduction of the enlarged bone or bones, and the operation may have to be repeated if growth continues.

Cherubism is a rare disorder characterised by painless enlargement of both sides of the mandible, which usually develops between 2 and 4 years. The condition runs a benign course and the swellings often regress a few years later.

54

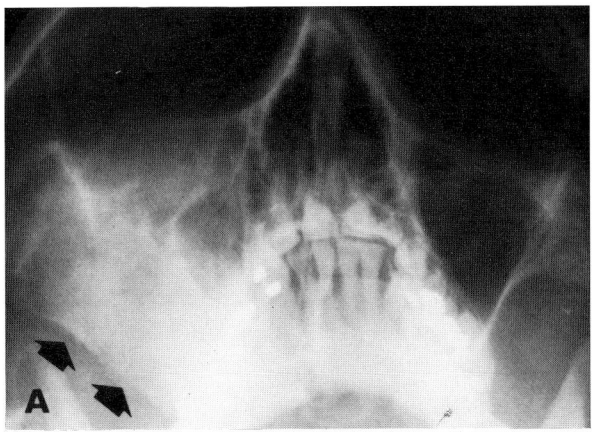

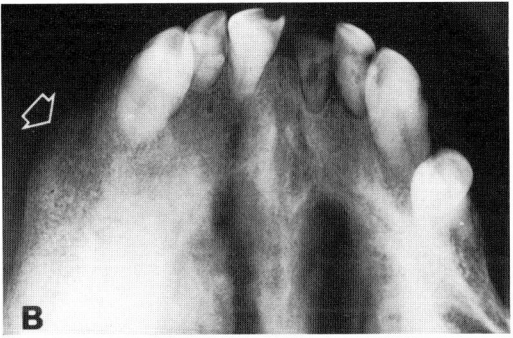

Fig. 7.1 Fibrous dysplasia of the lateral wall and floor of the right maxillary sinus. The bone is expanded and shows dense homogeneous opacification (arrowed). This feature is sometimes described as the 'ground glass' appearance. **B.** Intra-oral film of fibrous dysplasia in the right maxilla of a different case. There is thickening of the individual trabeculae resulting in an 'orange peel' appearance.

There is a *family history* in most cases, which suggests that it is transmitted as an autosomal dominant.[3] The pathological classification is uncertain, but it is usually considered to be a type of fibrous dysplasia.

Radiologically there are expanding multilocular radiolucent areas on both sides of the mandible, with absence of the developing teeth in the radiolucent areas.

OSSIFYING FIBROMA

The ossifying fibroma is a rare lesion which has more in common with fibrous dysplasia than neoplasia.[2] It seems to be a different entity from the similarly named tumour which occurs elsewhere in the skeleton.

Like fibrous dysplasia, it usually presents in adolescence or early adult life.

Radiologically it begins as an expanding radiolucent lesion, which may have a corticated margin and which often erodes the roots of adjacent teeth without displacing them. Dense areas of calcification soon develop within the radiolucency (Fig. 7.2) and can coalesce until the lesion becomes completely radio-opaque.

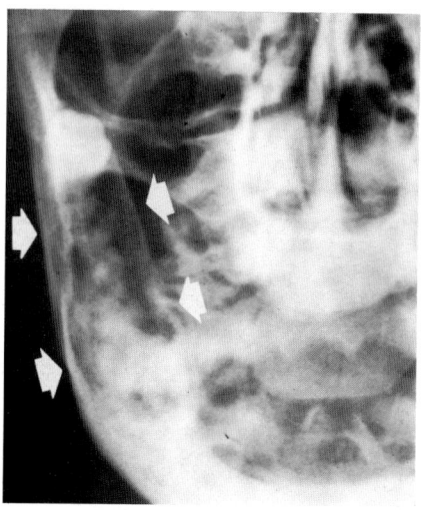

Fig. 7.2 Partially calcified ossifying fibroma expanding the right ramus of the mandible (arrowed).

The condition is undoubtedly benign and treatment is usually limited to surgical reduction of the expanded bone with a view to obtaining a good cosmetic result. Recurrence is common after surgery and subsequent reduction after a period of years may be necessary.

CEMENTOMA AND HYPERCEMENTOSIS

A **cementoma** is a mass of cementum which develops in the tooth bearing part of the maxilla or mandible. These lesions are initially radiolucent, but soon develop irregular areas of calcification and eventually become densely calcified. They are often multiple (Fig. 7.3) and can cause expansion of the overlying cortex when they become indistinguishable from fibrous dysplasia. They are said to be more common in negro than in other races.

Hypercementosis (cemental hyperplasia) is an asymptomatic

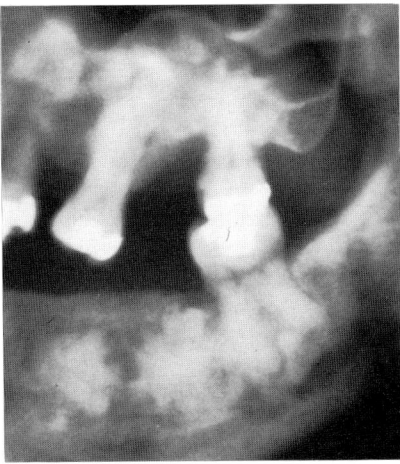

Fig. 7.3 Multiple cementomas of the maxilla and mandible showing as ill-defined opacities surrounded by a radiolucent margin in some places.

abnormality which can develop at any time in adult life. The aetiology is unknown. It often affects several adjacent teeth and appears radiologically as marked widening of the apical part of the root, with preservation of the radiolucent periodontal membrane *outside* the bulbous root (Fig. 7.4). The condition can be distinguished

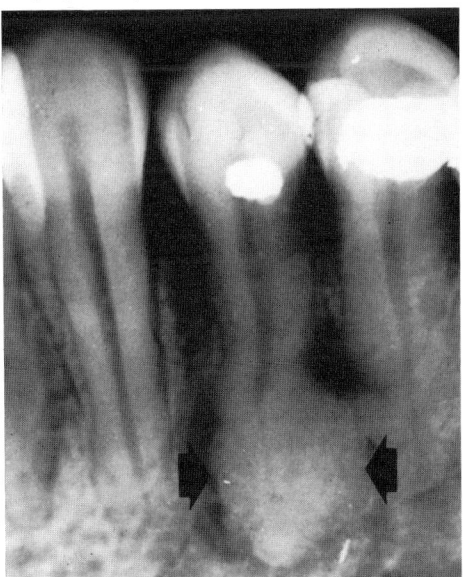

Fig. 7.4 Hypercementosis of ⎣4̄. There is a mass of cementum around the root (arrowed) giving it a bulbous appearance.

radiologically from a cementoma and from the hypercementosis of Paget's disease, as the dense calcification in these conditions lies outside the periodontal membrane in the trabecular bone.

PAGET'S DISEASE

Paget's disease affects the maxilla more frequently than the mandible and is usually bilateral. Most cases are preceded by Paget's disease of the skull vault.

As in other bones, the earliest radiological features are expansion and a loss of normal trabeculae. The trabeculae which remain behind become thickened, which results in the characteristic coarse trabecular pattern. Areas of dense bone sclerosis may develop later and in the tooth-bearing parts of the jaws, masses of cementum may develop adjacent to the roots of teeth (hypercementosis) or in edentulous areas (multiple cementomas). These abnormalities are illustrated in Figure 7.5.

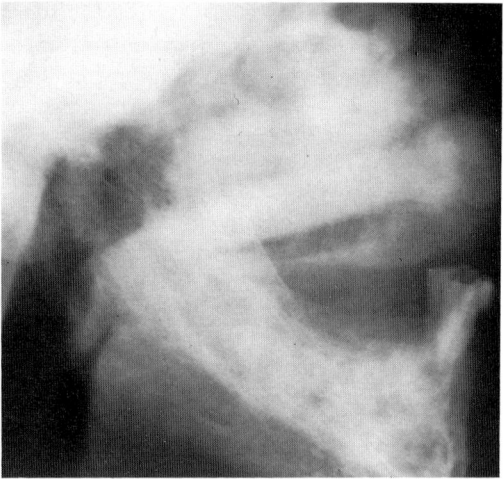

Fig. 7.5 Paget's disease of the maxilla and mandible. The maxilla is enlarged and contains coalescing areas of patchy sclerosis due to multiple cementoma. The mandible is expanded and has a coarse trabecular pattern with patchy sclerosis.

NON-NEOPLASTIC ACQUIRED CONDITIONS

Histiocytosis X[1] is the term used to describe three rare diseases which are characterised histiologically by a proliferation of mature histiocytes and radiologicaly by destructive lesions of bone which have well-defined but non-corticated margins. The most severe is *Letterer-Siwe disease,* which affects infants and which is often fatal. There are widespread skeletal radiolucencies and the skull vault is usually affected. *Hand-Schüller-Christian disease* is a more chronic disease of older children and adolescents which also results in large radiolucencies in the skull vault and which can affect the alveolar bone so that the teeth seem to 'float' in the soft tissues. *Eosinophilic granuloma* of bone occurs in young adults and often runs a benign self-limiting course. The lesions are usually solitary and often develop in the skull vault or mandible (Fig. 7.6). In the early stages there is no cortical margin but one can develop if the lesion stops growing or regresses.

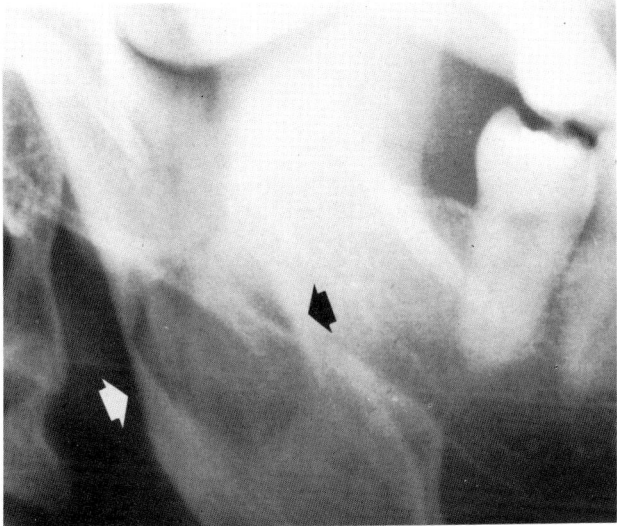

Fig. 7.6 Histiocytosis X showing as a non-corticated but well-defined defect (arrowed) in the trabecular pattern of the ramus of the mandible.

The brown tumour of *hyperparathyroidism* occasionally occurs in the jaws, and appears as an expanding radiolucent area with an ill defined margin and with erosion of the roots of adjacent teeth (Fig. 7.7). Hyperparathyroidism may also result in widespread resorption of the lamina dura of all the teeth, and if this unique radiological abnormality is present, the diagnosis can be made with complete confidence. Chronic renal failure[1] can result in similar changes but, like renal osteodystrophy in other bones, also causes patchy sclerosis.

Midline granuloma is a very rare destructive lesion of the hard palate, which appears radiologically as a poorly defined radiolucent area. It can be associated with granulomata in the nose and with more widespread granulomata in the lungs and kidneys (*Wegener's granulomatosis*).

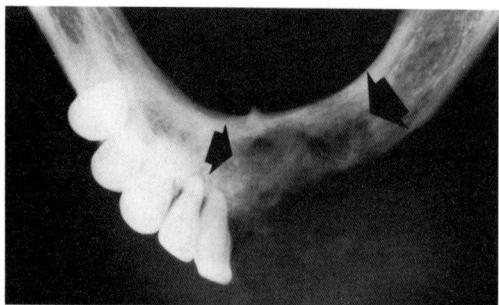

Fig. 7.7   Brown tumour of hyperparathyroidism. There is an irregular defect in the anterior part of the mandible (arrowed).

REFERENCES

1. Kelly W H, et al 1980 Radiographic changes of the jawbones in end stage renal disease. Oral Surgery 50: 372–381
2. Langdon J D, Rapidis A D, Patel M F 1976 Ossifying fibroma — one disease or six? An analysis of 39 fibro-osseus lesions of the jaws. British Journal of Oral Surgery 14: 1–11
3. Peters W 1979 Cherubism: a study of 20 cases from one family. Journal of Oral Surgery 47: 307
4. Rapidis A D, Langdon J D, Patel M F, Harvey P W 1979 Histiocytosis X. British Journal of Oral Surgery 16: 219–233
5. Schmamon A, Smith I, Ackerman L V 1970 Benign fibro-osseus lesions of the mandible and maxilla. Cancer 26: 303–312

8

Osteomyelitis, infective and inflammatory bone conditions

PYOGENIC INFECTIONS

Acute pyogenic osteomyelitis is usually precipitated by local conditions, such as peri-apical dental infections, dental extractions or a fracture. Considering the frequency of peri-apical infection, osteomyelitis is surprisingly rare. It commonly affects the mandible and is almost unknown in the maxilla. The infecting organism is usually *Streptococcus* or *Staphylococcus*.

Acute osteomyelitis in children may complicate severe infections such as measles and typhoid, and is presumably a blood-borne infection in these cases. It may also be a complication of local pyogenic infections such as tonsillitis. Osteomyelitis is more common in systemic conditions such as malnutrition, diabetes mellitus, leucopenia and sickle cell anaemia. The incidence of infection is higher after radiotherapy and in osteopetrosis.

The radiological abnormalities do not appear until the clinical symptoms of pain, tenderness and soft tissue swelling have been present for a few days. The earliest change is an ill-defined area of rarefaction in the trabecular bone, or rarefaction of the lamina dura of a recently extracted tooth.

The rarefaction rapidly progresses to more extensive bone destruction with resorption of the lamina dura of adjacent teeth (Fig. 8.1). *Subperiosteal new bone* always develops, but may be difficult to demonstrate unless multiple radiographs are taken in different projections (Figs 8.2, 8.3).

The treatment is prolonged antibiotics, with surgical decortication in all but the earliest cases.

Sequestra are common if the appropriate antibiotics are not given at an early stage and appear as opacities lying in cavities. A pathological fracture may occur if the mandible is seriously weakened (Fig. 8.4).

Chronic osteomyelitis[1] may follow acute osteomyelitis and has similar radiological features, with patchy osteoporosis, patchy sclerosis

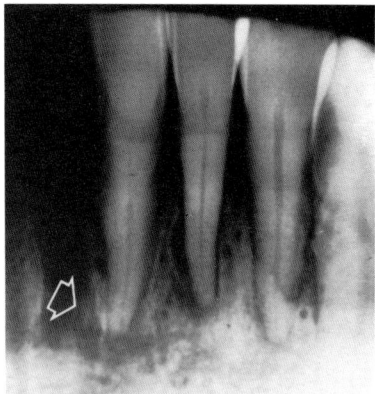

Fig. 8.1   Early osteomyelitis of the mandible due to recent extraction of 2̄1̄. There is a defect in the lamina dura around the socket of the extracted tooth (arrowed) and patchy osteoporosis in the adjacent bone.

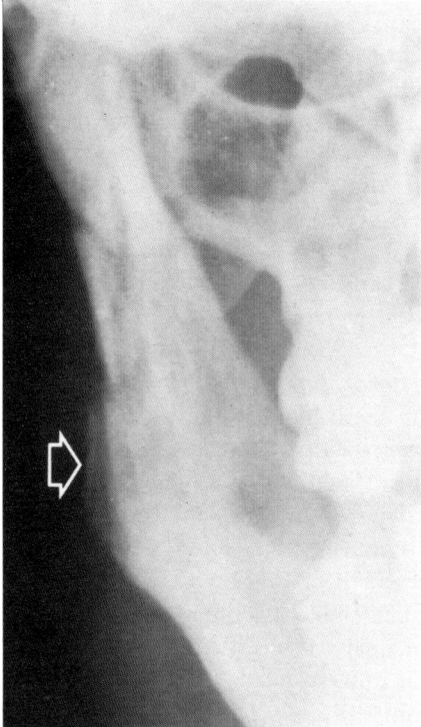

Fig. 8.2   Osteomyelitis of the body and ramus of the mandible with sub-periosteal new bone laterally (arrowed).

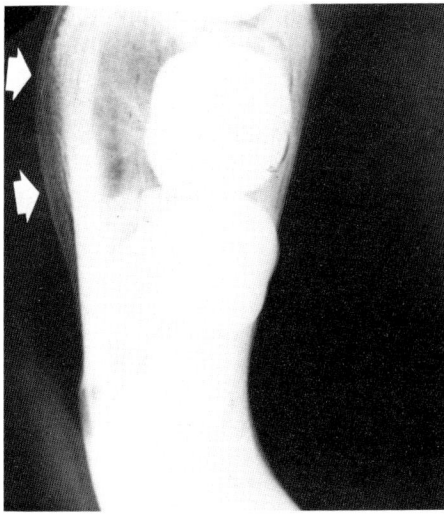

Fig. 8.3 Occlusal view of the mandible of an 8-year-old child showing bone rarefaction and sub-periosteal new bone formation (arrowed) lateral to 6̄⌋. These abnormalities, which are typical of pyogenic osteomyelitis, were not visible on the PA, OPG or lateral films.

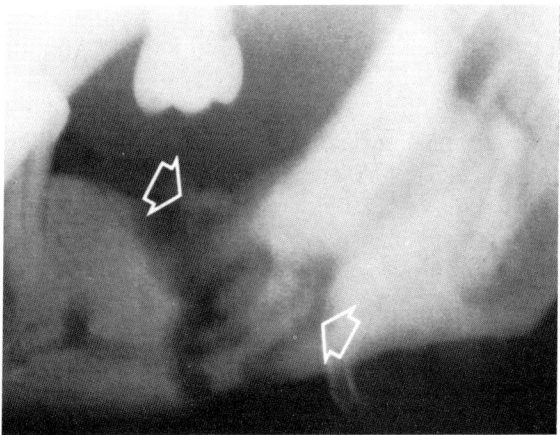

Fig. 8.4 Chronic osteomyelitis with large and small sequestra (arrowed) plus a pathological fracture through the body of the mandible.

and sequestra lying in cavities. However, sub-periosteal new bone is less common.

Garre's osteomyelitis[4] (sub-periosteal osteomyelitis) presents as a tender bony swelling with intra-oral sinuses. The infecting organisms are usually Gram-positive cocci, which suggest that it is a sub-acute form of pyogenic osteomyelitis and not a separate pathological entity. The dominant radiological feature is the formation of dense sub-periosteal new bone. There is also patchy sclerosis in the underlying bone, patchy rarefaction and sequestrum formation.

Osteoradionecrosis is the name given to a particularly intractable form of chronic osteomyelitis, which is an occasional sequel to radiotherapy. Radiotherapy itself rarely produces any radiological change in the trabecular pattern of the maxilla or mandible, but very high doses occasionally result in rarefaction or sclerosis. The radiological abnormalities produced by infection are widespread patchy sclerosis, with areas of rarefaction and multiple sequestra. The disease often spreads throughout the mandible and is extremely difficult to control with antibiotics. Hyperbaric oxygen seems to be effective in some cases.

Osteomyelitis in infants is an uncommon infection and is probably of haematogenous origin, as it appears during the first three months of life before the teeth have erupted. Clinically it presents as an acute systemic illness with fever and gastrointestinal upset. It is much more common in the maxilla than in the mandible. Radiologically, there is extensive destruction of bone, with exfoliation of the developing teeth, sequestrum formation and occasional sub-periosteal new bone. The differential diagnosis in the mandible is infantile cortical hyperostosis. It can result in partial anodontia due to loss of developing teeth and to permanent asymmetry of the mandible if the infection destroys the epiphyseal cartilage of the condylar neck.

NON-PYOGENIC INFECTIONS

Condensing osteitis is a rare, low grade infection of alveolar bone, which can result from chronic peri-apical or periodontal infection. The characteristic radiological abnormality is an irregularly defined area of dense sclerosis around a peri-apical radiolucency, or a deep periodontal pocket. The sclerosis often persists after removal of the responsible tooth or teeth and is one cause of a bone island. Radiologically it is very similar to peri-apical osteopetrosis and the two conditions may be indistinguishable.

The condition is often asymptomatic and is usually self-limiting. Antibiotics are occasionally prescribed.

Actinomycosis[3] is essentially a soft tissue infection, but cervico-facial actinomycosis occasionally spreads to the mandible and results in chronic osteomyelitis, with patchy rarefaction and sclerosis.

Tuberculous osteomyelitis[6] occurs rarely and is usually a sequel to dental extractions in a patient with open tuberculous. Radiologically it appears as an irregular area of bone destruction.

Tertiary syphilis[7] can result in a gumma (commonly in the hard palate) or in a low-grade osteomyelitis. Radiologically these lesions are destructive, with little new bone formation.

NON-INFECTIVE INFLAMMATORY BONE CONDITIONS

Peri-apical osteopetrosis[2] (focal peri-apical osteopetrosis, osteosclerosis) is an inflammatory condition of unknown aetiology, which affects the alveolar bone adjacent to the roots of vital and non-vital teeth. It can begin as a radiolucent area, but this soon progresses to an area of dense sclerosis, which can be larger than the original radiolucency. The condition is more common posteriorly than anteriorly and the abnormalities may be multiple. Small sclerotic areas may coalesce to produce larger areas measuring up to 1 cm in diameter. The margins are usually irregular. The sclerosis persists after extraction of the teeth and is therefore seen in edentulous areas. Radiologically it is similar to condensing osteitis and the two conditions are often indistinguishable. It is one cause of a bone island.

The condition is self-limiting and seems to be asymptomatic. No treatment is required, but biopsy is sometimes carried out to exclude low grade infection or neoplasm.

Caffey's disease (infantile cortical hyperostosis) affects the mandible in most infants who develop the disease and is characterised radiologically by sub-periosteal new bone formation during the first five months of life (Fig. 8.5).

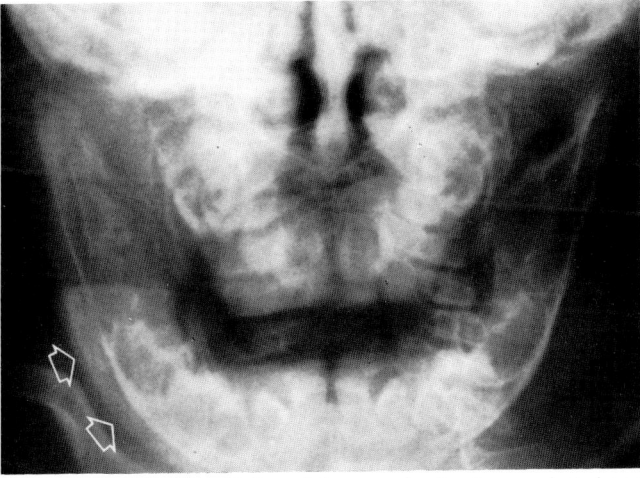

Fig. 8.5 Caffey's disease in an infant of three months showing a periosteal reaction on the right side of the mandible (arrowed). The crowns of the developing deciduous teeth are just beginning to calcify in the radiolucent dental crypts.

It can also affect other bones, particularly the ribs, clavicles, radii and ulnae. The sub-periosteal new bone is gradually resorbed during the following months, but may not resorb completely. Mandibular asymmetry during infancy is a common sequel and can persist into adolescence and adult life, with malocclusion of the teeth.

The differential diagnosis is pyogenic osteomyelitis and, in premature infants, rickets.[5]

REFERENCES

1. Daromola J O, Ajagbe H A 1982 Chronic osteomyelitis of the mandible in adults: a study of 34 cases. British Journal of Oral Surgery 20: 58–62
2. Eversole L R, Stone C E, Strub D 1984 Focal sclerosing osteomyelitis/focal peri-apical osteopetrosis: radiographic patterns. Oral Surgery, Oral Medicine, Oral Pathology 58: 456–460
3. Fradis M, Zisman D, Podoshin L, Wellisch G 1976 Actinomycosis of the face and neck. Acta Otolaryngology 102: 87–89
4. Johannsen A 1977 Chronic sclerosing osteomyelitis of the mandible: radiographic differential diagnosis from fibrous dysplasia. Acta Radiologica: Diagnosis 18: 360–368
5. Thomas P S 1978 The 'Mandibular Mantle': a sign of rickets in very low birth weight infants. British Journal of Radiology 51: 93–98
6. Worsaae N, Reibel J, Rechnitzer C 1984 Tuberculous osteomyelitis of the mandible. British Journal of Oral Surgery 22: 93–98
7. Yusuf H, Battacharya M N 1982 Syphilitic osteomyelitis of the mandible. British Journal of Oral Surgery 20: 122–128

9

Developmental abnormalities of the maxilla and mandible

LOCALISED

The Stafne bone cavity is a round or oval corticated defect in the posterior part of the mandible below the inferior dental canal (Fig. 9.1). The cortical outline is usually complete, but may be defective inferiorly where it is continuous with the inferior border of the mandible. The abnormality is probably present at birth and is invariably asymptomatic. It can contain part of the submandibular salivary gland.[1]

A dental crypt containing an uncalcified tooth germ is a normal appearance in a child, but is occasionally misdiagnosed as a cyst or tumour, particularly in the lower molar region. (Fig. 9.2).

Idiopathic sclerosis (bone islands; enostosis) are terms used to describe areas of bone sclerosis which appear in the tooth bearing parts of the maxilla and mandible after childhood. They may be single (Fig.

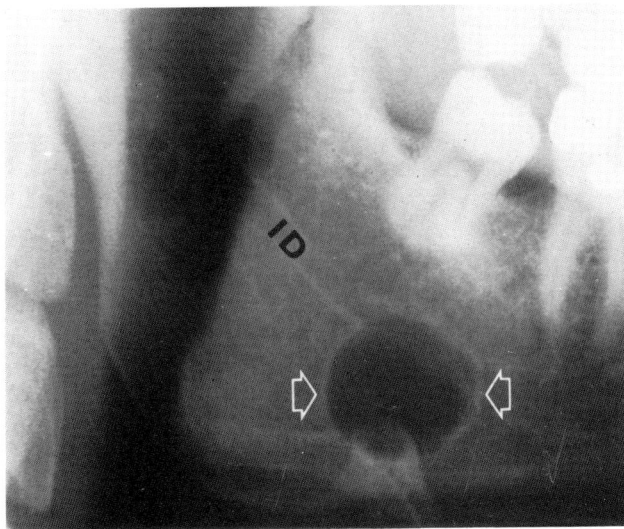

Fig. 9.1 Stafne bone cavity with the characteristic appearance of a corticated defect in the posterior part of the mandible below the inferior dental canal (ID).

67

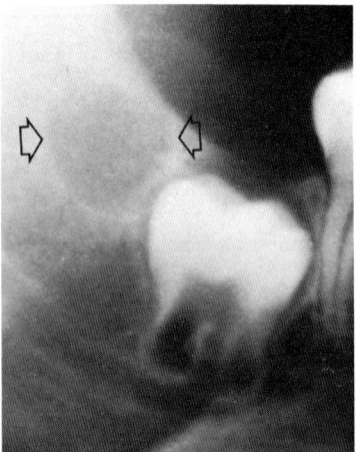

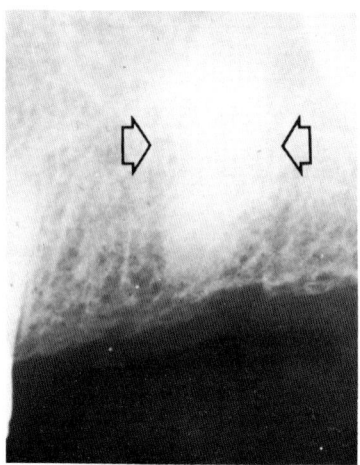

Fig. 9.2 Normal dental crypt (arrowed) containing the uncalcified tooth germ of a developing 8̅| in a 9-year-old child.

Fig. 9.3 Idiopathic bone sclerosis (bone island) in the upper left premolar region (confirmed histologically).

9.3), or multiple and can be quite extensive,[2] particularly in the mandible. The margin is usually irregular, but can be smooth. A bone island may result from condensing osteitis or peri-apical osteopetrosis, but most cases are idiopathic. Although the condition is common, it is sometimes necessary to perform a biopsy to confirm the diagnosis and exlude low-grade infection or a sclerotic tumour.

Torus palatinus and torus mandibularis are common non-neoplastic bony outgrowths which develop in adults of all ages. Radiologically there is progressive thickening of the cortex, due to laying down of sub-periosteal lamellar bone. Torus palatinus arises from the midline of the hard palate posteriorly and torus mandibularis, which is usually bilateral, arises from the inner tables of the mandible in the premolar region (Fig. 9.4). They are sometimes mistaken for ivory osteomas, which they resemble radiologically, but their anatomical position should indicate the diagnosis. They are occasionally removed or reduced in size if they make it impossible to fit satisfactory dentures.

Condylar hyperplasia is a rare condition of unknown aetiology, which develops at puberty and which is always unilateral. There is generalised enlargement of the condylar head of the mandible which is often misdiagnosed as a bone tumour. The unilateral growth results in the midline of the mandible being displaced to the unaffected side and in an open bite on the affected side (Fig. 9.5).

Bilateral coronoid hyperplasia is another rare abnormality of growth, which limits mandibular opening as the large coronoid processes impinge against the

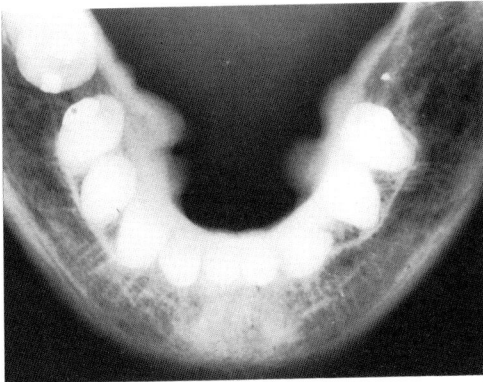

Fig. 9.4 Bilateral torus mandibularis. There are two localised areas of thickening of the inner tables of the mandible in the premolar regions.

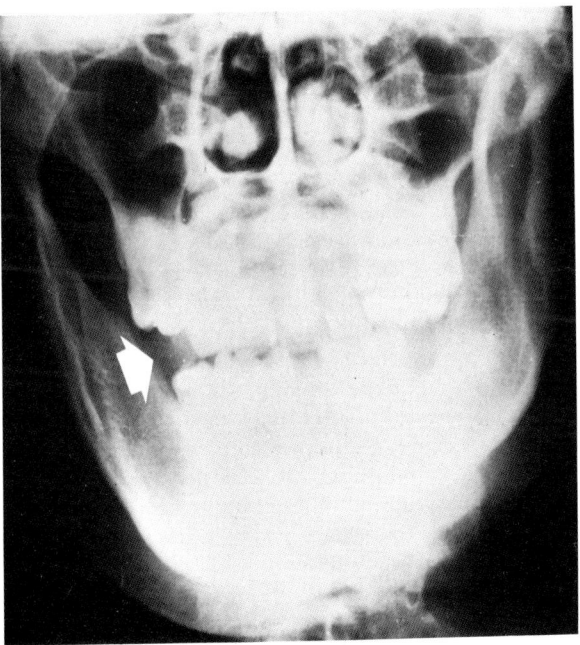

Fig. 9.5 Hyperplasia of the right mandibular condyle with an open bite on the right side (arrowed).

zygomatic arches (unilateral coronoid enlargement is usually due to an osteochondroma).

FACE AND SKULL

Cleft palate is the most common developmental anomaly of the maxillo-facial region. The diagnosis is clinical and should be made at birth. If the cleft extends anteriorly through the alveoar bone on one or both sides, there will be displacement of the upper anterior teeth and occasional absence of the lateral incisors. The maxilla often fails to grow normally during childhood, which results in relative mandibular protrusion in adult life.

In the *Pierre Robin Syndrome* the mandible is extremely small, resulting in a 'bird face' deformity. The larynx is usually underdeveloped and cleft palate is common.

Hypertelorism (Greig's ocular hypertelorism) is recognised clinically by the wide space between the eyes. It may be accompanied by incomplete development of the alveolar arches of the maxilla, with subsequent malocclusion in adult life, and by partial anodontia of the maxillary teeth.

In the *Treacher–Collins syndrome* (mandibulo-facial dysostosis, first arch dysplasia) the striking facial abnormalities are the anti-mongoloid tilt of the eyes, small deformed ears and a small mandible. Radiologically the zygomatic arches are absent or incomplete, and there is underdevelopment of the maxilla and of the mandible.

Unilateral condylar hypoplasia can occur as a spontaneous abnormality, but in most cases there is a history of trauma or infection during childhood which could have damaged the epiphyseal cartilage of the condylar neck. The degree of facial deformity depends upon the age when normal epiphyseal growth stops. In a severe case the condylar head is small and the condylar neck absent. The joint space is often narrowed and bony ankylosis is occasionally seen. The ramus of the mandible is short and the gonial angle greatly increased. The occlusal plane of the posterior teeth is elevated and the midline of the mandible and maxilla is deviated to the affected side.

Bilateral condylar hypoplasia occasionally occurs as a spontaneous abnormality and is a rare sequel to injury or infection, but most cases are associated with more wide-spread developmental abnormalities such as the Treacher–Collins syndrome, the Pierre Robin syndrome and arthrogryphosis multiplex congenita. In most cases the condylar heads are small and the condylar necks virtually absent. The temporo-mandibular joint spaces are usually narrowed and are occasionally ankylosed (see Fig. 14.8). The rami are extremely short, the gonial angles greatly increased and the whole mandible is underdeveloped, producing the characteristic 'bird face' deformity,

Crouzon's disease (cranio-facial dysostosis) results in occular hypertelorism with underdevelopment of the maxilla, leading to relative mandibular protrusion. The nose has a characteristic 'parrot beak' appearance and there is usually craniostenosis of some or all of the skull sutures.

GENERALISED

These rare conditions are often due to an autosomal dominant gene, so there is frequently a history of similarly affected relatives.

Cleido-cranial dysostosis affects the development of bones which ossify from membrane and the teeth. There are always multiple dental abnormalities, the principal ones being prolonged retention of the deciduous teeth, failure of their permanent successors to erupt, abnormally shaped teeth, supernumary teeth and partial anodontia (Fig. 9.6).

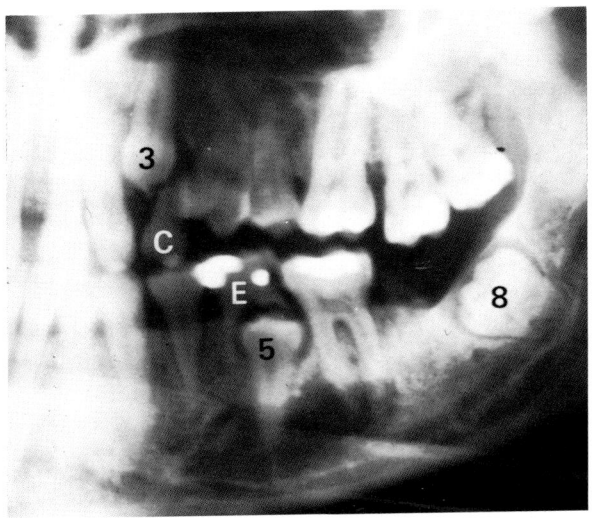

Fig. 9.6 Non-eruption of three permanent teeth (numbered) with prolonged retention of two deciduous teeth (lettered) in an adult with cleidocranial dysostosis.

Skull x-rays show often fontanelles in adult life and multiple Wormian bones at the sutures. The clavicles are absent or underdeveloped, the scapulae are small, the ribs are short and angled downwards, and the pubic symphysis remains open in adult life.

Achondroplasia affects the bones which ossify from cartilage; consequently the maxilla is underdeveloped and this results in relative mandibular protrusion in adult life. Eruption of the maxillary teeth is often delayed and there is frequently malocclusion of the teeth which have erupted. The most significant abnormalities occur in the long bones, lumbar spine and pelvis resulting in dwarfism, spinal stenosis and lumbar lordosis.

Multiple neurofibromatosis (von Recklinghausen's disease) can result in asymmetrical growth of the facial bones and in localised bone defects.[3]

In *Gorlin's Syndrome* (multiple basal cell naevi syndrome) multiple odontogenic keratocysts develop in the maxilla and mandible during childhood. The more significant abnormality is the development of multiple basal cell carcinomas, which begin to develop during the second decade. Bifid ribs are common.

Gardner's syndrome (Fitzgerald–Gardner syndrome) is a variant of familial polyposis of the colon and is accompanied by multiple ivory osteomas of the skull and facial bones, including the mandible.

Albers-Schönberg disease (osteopetrosis, marble bone disease) results in generalised bone sclerosis, which affects the maxillofacial region as well as the rest of the skeleton. In addition, there is thickening of the lamina dura around the teeth and an increased susceptibility to osteomyelitis of the mandible after dental extractions.

In *Hurler's Syndrome* (gargoylism) the articular surface of the condyle is usually concave instead of convex and this abnormality is specific for the syndrome.

Acromegaly results in continued growth of the facial bones, including the alveolar arches, and this results in gradual spacing of the teeth. The mandible grows more than the maxilla, which can result in gross mandibular protrusion (Fig. 9.7). The pituitary fossa is enlarged, the skull vault is thickened and there

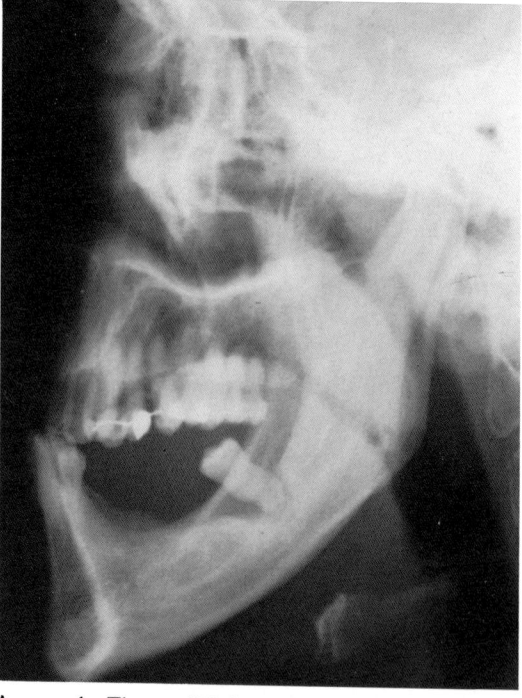

Fig. 9.7 Acromegaly. The mandible is excessively large, resulting in mandibular protrusion and malocclusion. There are spaces between some of the upper teeth due to continued maxillary growth. The pituitary fossa is enlarged.

is often enlargement of the frontal sinuses. The tongue is sometimes enlarged, and this can be shown on a lateral film of the facial bones.

REFERENCES

1. Adra N A, Barakat N, Melhem R E 1980 Salivary gland inclusions in the mandible: Stafne's idiopathic bone cavity. American Journal of Roentgenology 134: 1082–1083
2. Bhaskar S N 1968 Multiple enostosis: report of 16 cases. Journal of Oral Surgery 26: 321–326
3. Gupta S K 1979 The radiological features of craniofacial neurofibromatosis: Clinical Radiology 30: 553–557

10

Abnormalities of eruption and resorption

IMPACTION AND ABNORMAL ERUPTION DUE TO LOCAL CONDITIONS

A tooth is said to be *impacted* if it is physically prevented from erupting by dense bone, another tooth, or an odontome. The teeth most commonly affected are the lower third molars and upper canines because they erupt late into the dental arches and have to fit into spaces of limited size. The upper third molars, lower second premolars and lower canines are occasionally impacted.

The lower third molar erupts 5–6 years after the lower second molar and the space between the second molar and the anterior border of the ramus of the mandible may be less than the size of its crown. The tooth may impact horizontally, vertically or obliquely and it may be erupted or partially erupted (Figs 10.1, 10.2, 10.3). An unerupted third molar which is impacted against the roots of a second molar occasionally causes root resorption.

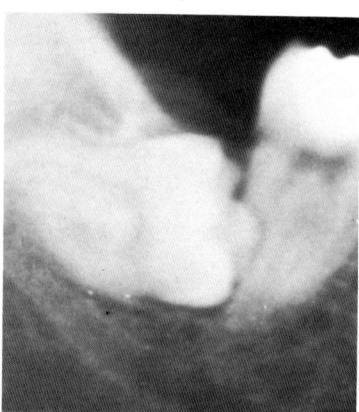 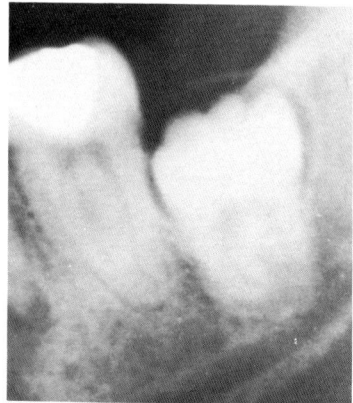

Fig. 10.1 Horizontal impaction of ⁻8̄|.

Fig. 10.2 Vertical impaction of⁻8̄ . There is an irregular area of bone rarefaction around the roots of ⁻6̄ which is typical of an alveolar abscess.

74

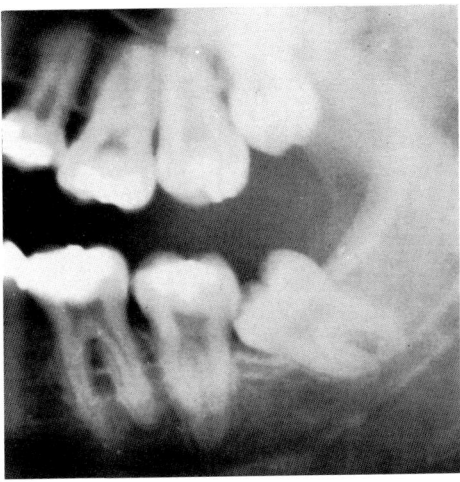

Fig. 10.3   Mesio-angular impaction of $\overline{|8.}$

Pericoronitis is almost inevitable if an impacted lower third molar is partially erupted and recurrent attacks can result in local bone resorption in the absence of serious bone infection (osteomyelitis). Partially erupted third molars can precipitate local periodontal disease and often develop extensive caries (see Fig. 2.4).

The upper canine erupts 2–3 years after the second incisor and first premolar and, if space between these teeth is too small, the canine will impact, usually obliquely (Fig. 10.4). Its relationship to the dental arch is best shown on a true vertex occlusal film. An impacted canine can resorb the roots of adjacent teeth, particularly the second incisor, and a dentigerous cyst may develop around the crown. It may erupt late in life after the normally erupted upper teeth have been extracted and can result in acute pericoronitis.

Supernumary and supplemental teeth often become impacted (see Figs 4.6, 4.7) and are a rare cause of normally developed teeth becoming impacted.

Fibro-osseus lesions, cysts and tumours can delay or prevent the eruption of normal teeth.

A *cleft palate* which extends through the dental arch usually delays or prevents the eruption of the upper second incisor and canine teeth.

ABNORMAL ERUPTION DUE TO SYSTEMIC CONDITIONS

A few permanent teeth will sometimes fail to erupt in the absence of any local or generalised abnormality. There is frequently a family history of

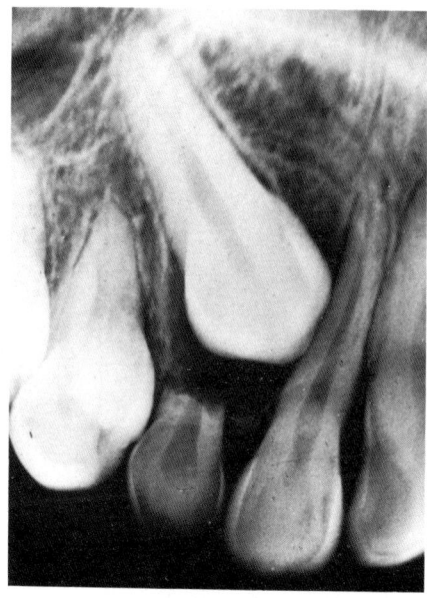

Fig. 10.4   Oblique impaction of 3⌋. There is physiological resorption of the root of
C⌋.

this condition in affected individuals, which suggests that it is
transmitted as an autosomal dominant.

Cleido-cranial dysostosis (see Fig. 9.6) and *achondroplasia* are often associated
with delayed eruption and non-eruption of the permanent teeth.

Eruption depends on normal circulating *levels of thyroxine and growth
hormone.* It is therefore delayed in hypopituitarism and hypothyroidism and is
premature in patients with gigantism. Eruption is late in progeria.

PHYSIOLOGICAL RESORPTION

Resorption of the roots of deciduous teeth is normal and most of the
root structure is usually resorbed before the tooth is lost (Fig. 10.5).
There can be extensive resorption of the crown with the formation of a
'pink spot' clinically.

If the permanent successor is absent, the root of the deciduous tooth
may become ankylosed to the alveolar bone and its occlusal surface
eventually becomes submerged below the levels of the occlusal surfaces
of the adjacent permanent teeth.

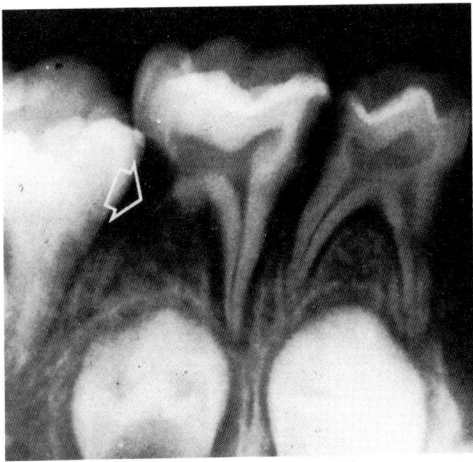

Fig. 10.5   Physiological resorption of the distal root of E̅| (arrowed).

EXTERNAL RESORPTION

Unerupted teeth may become resorbed after a period of years. The process usually affects the dentine of the root, but the enamel is occasionally affected (Fig. 10.6).

Root-treated and non-vital teeth are sometimes resorbed. The process usually begins at the apex of the root, but can start laterally.

Traumatised teeth are often subject to root resorption (Ch. 11). It can occur after root fracture or partial avulsion and is a common sequel to reimplantation after complete avulsion.

Surgical reimplantation is usually followed by root resorption. It seems to make little difference if the tooth has been root treated and a

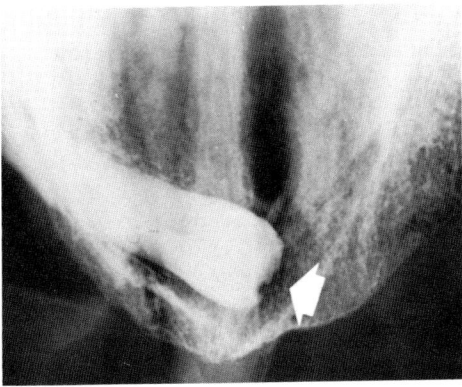

Fig. 10.6   Resorption of the enamel of an unerupted canine in an elderly edentulous patient (arrowed).

recent paper stated that over 60% of reimplanted canine teeth showed evidence of root resorption within 2 years.[1]

Idiopathic resorption is usually external and may affect one tooth or several adjacent teeth. It usually commences at the root apex, but can start just below the gingival margin (Fig. 10.7).

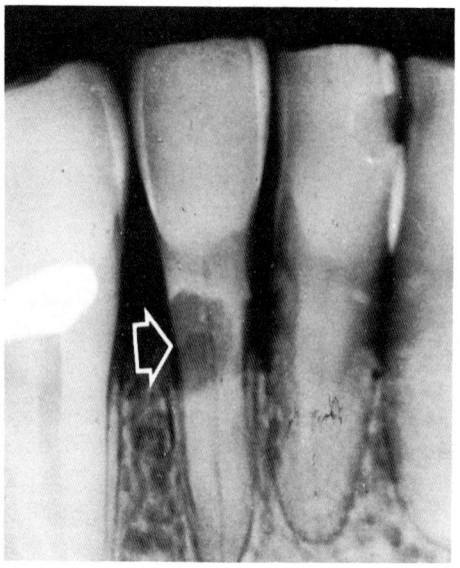

Fig. 10.7 Idiopathic external resorption of the root of the 2| (arrowed).

Radiologically external resorption in these cases is always preceded by local bone resorption. The progress of root resorption is often intermittent, with periods of months or years when no resorption takes place and the process may arrest completely with the development of normal trabecular bone and a normal lamina dura around the partially resorbed root.

Chronic infection, fibro-osseus lesions and malignant tumours can cause root resorption and occasionally displace the roots of the affected teeth.

Simple cysts, benign tumours and impacted teeth can also cause root resorption and usually displace the roots of the affected teeth (see Fig. 5.4).

INTERNAL RESORPTION

Internal root resorption is usually idiopathic, but can be a sequal to trauma. Radiologically there is localised expansion of the pulp chamber or pulp canal, which can enlarge until the soft tissues of the pulp are continuous with the periodontal membrane (Fig. 10.8).

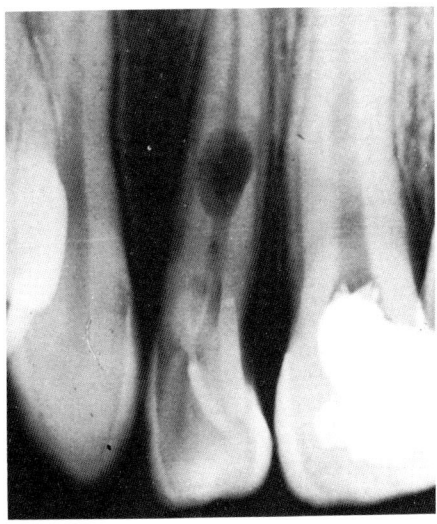

Fig. 10.8 Idiopathic internal resorption of the root of 2|. There is dens invaginatus (dens in dente) deforming the crown.

REFERENCES

1. Hall G M, Reade P C 1983 Root resorption associated with autotransplanted maxillary teeth. British Journal of Oral and Maxillofacial Surgery 21: 179–191

11

Dental trauma

FRACTURES OF TEETH

Fractures of the teeth are caused by direct trauma to the crown and occur most frequently in the upper incisor region. They are common in children and are usually due to a fall. The cause in adults is more likely to be a road traffic accident, a sporting activity or an assault.

A fracture of the crown should be obvious clinically, but fractured teeth should always be radiographed (Fig. 11.1) as there may be a second fracture involving the root. Fractures of the crown which enter the pulp chamber will invariably result in infective pulpitis and pulp death, unless pulp capping is carried out at an early stage. Detached fragments of the crown may be driven into the adjacent soft tissues such as the lips and soft tissue radiographs of these areas should be taken if this is suspected.

Root fractures are also caused by trauma to the crown. They are usually single and transverse (Fig. 11.2), but can be multiple. Oblique

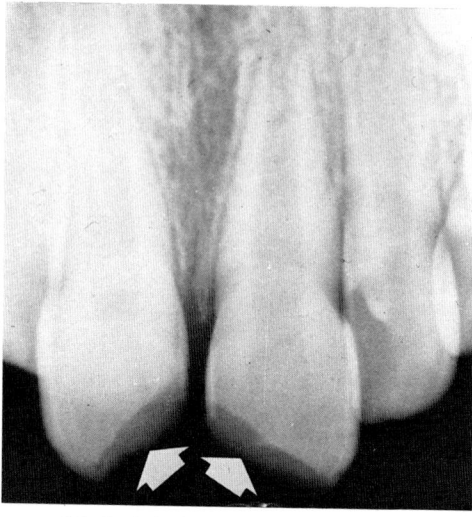

Fig. 11.1   Fractures of the incisal edges of the crowns of $\underline{1}|$ and $|\underline{1}$ (arrowed).

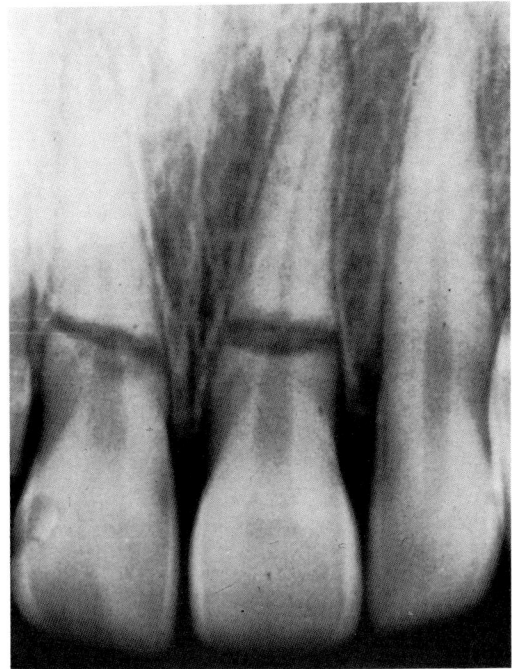

Fig. 11.2   Fractures of the roots of 1⌋ and ⌊1.

fractures which extend into the oral cavity will inevitably cause infective pulpitis and pulp death. Root fractures show best on intra-oral non-screen dental film and may be invisible on extra-oral films.

Root resorption is a common sequel to root fracture. The process usually begins as a localised area of bone rarefaction at the root apex and progresses intermittently over a period of years until the tooth becomes quite loose and has to be removed.

Attempted extraction may result in a fracture of the crown or root, especially in non-vital teeth, as dentine becomes more brittle after pulp death. Root fragments from upper molar teeth can be displaced into the maxillary sinus (Fig. 11.3). Small root fragments in alveolar bone are usually left behind as they rarely affect healing of the socket and do not seem to predispose to infection. They can be distinguished from small areas of bone sclerosis by the presence of a radiolucent root canal (Fig. 11.4).

AVULSION OF TEETH

Avulsion of teeth is more common in children than in adults and is usually seen in the upper incisor region.

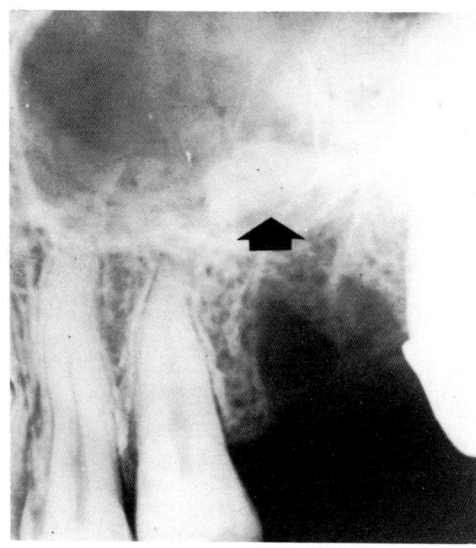

Fig. 11.3 Two roots (arrowed) of ⌊6 have been displaced into the left maxillary sinus in the course of an attempted extraction.

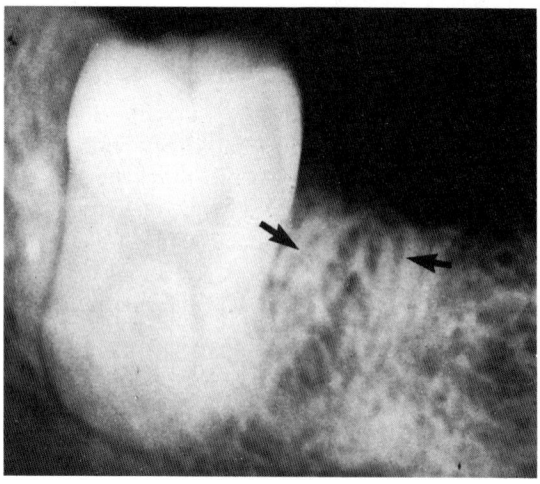

Fig. 11.4 Root fragments resulting from incomplete extraction of 7⌉ some years earlier. The root canals are just visible (arrowed) as faint radiolucent lines.

Complete avulsion (Fig. 11.5A) should be obvious clinically, but the socket should always be radiographed to check for residual root fragments and to exclude the possibility of an associated fracture of the alveolar bone.

Partial avulsion is usually diagnosed clinically, often by the patient,

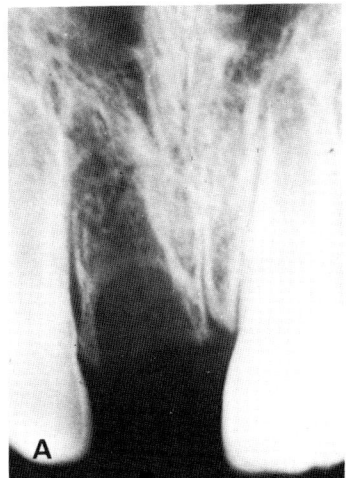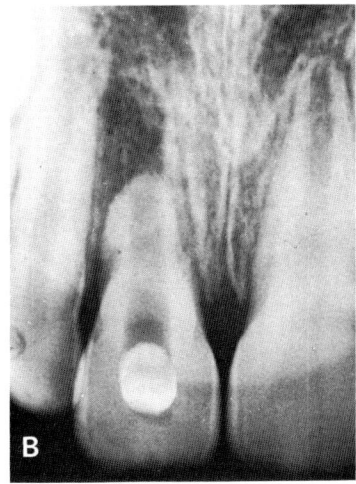

Fig. 11.5 A.   Complete avulsion of _1⌋_ in an 8-year-old child. **B.** Partial root resorption 6 months later, after re-implantation.

who will be aware of the sudden onset of malocclusion after severe trauma to the teeth. Radiographs may show widening of the periodontal membrane and small fractures of the lamina dura. Partial avulsion usually results in pulp death due to disruption of the neurovascular bundle at the root apex, and carries the risk of abscess formation if the tooth is not root-treated. Arrested growth often follows partial avulsion of a tooth with an incompletely developed root (Fig. 11.6).

Root resorption is a common sequel to partial avulsion (Fig. 11.7) and is extremely common after reimplantation of a completely avulsed tooth (Fig. 11.5B). The process usually begins at the root apex and is always preceded by a localised area of bone rarefaction. Resorption may be intermittent, with periods of months or years when no further resorption takes place and the process sometimes arrests completely with the formation of normal trabecular bone and a normal lamina dura around the partially resorbed root.

ALVEOLAR FRACTURES

Alveolar fractures are usually caused by *blunt trauma* on several adjacent teeth and are most common in the incisor region. The fracture lines can be difficult to detect and are best seen in intra-oral peri-apical or occlusal films. An alveolar fracture should always be suspected in a patient with a fracture of the teeth or facial bones.

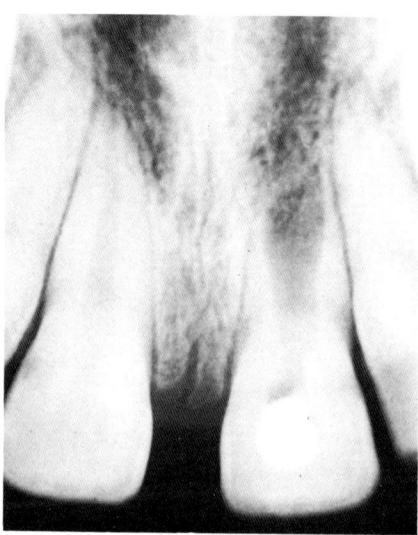

Fig. 11.6   Failure of normal root development of ⌊1 after partial avulsion 3 years earlier. The root apex is still wide open although the child is now aged 12 years.

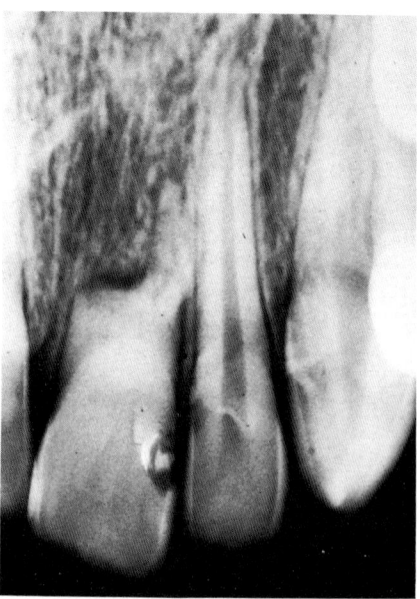

Fig. 11.7   Extensive resorption of the root of ⌊1 resulting from partial avulsion 18 months earlier, when the incisal edge of the crown had been fractured; the child is now aged 12 years.

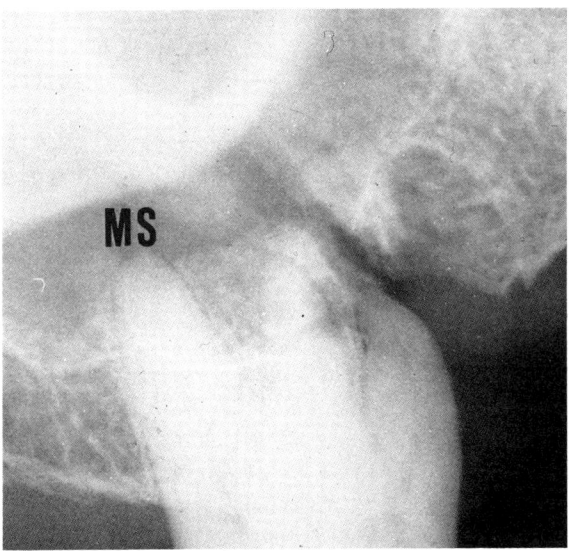

Fig. 11.8   Alveolar fracture extending into the maxillary sinus (MS) which resulted from the attempted extraction of 7|.

Attempted extraction can produce an alveolar fracture, particularly in the upper molar region of a patient with a large maxillary sinus (Fig. 11.8). Attempted extraction of a lower molar tooth occasionally fractures the thin lingual plate, with displacement of the tooth into the soft tissues of the floor of the mouth (Fig. 11.9).

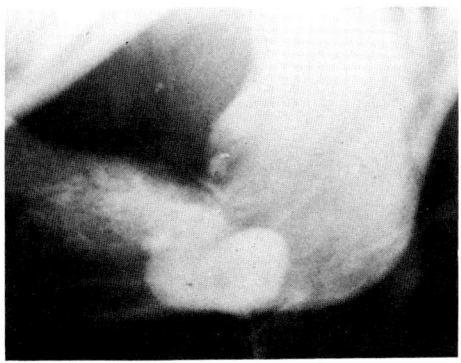

Fig. 11.9   Displacement of |8 into the soft tissues of the floor of the mouth following fracture of the lingual plate during attempted extraction.

12

Fractures of the mandible

CLASSIFICATION

Fractures of the mandible are classified according to the site of the fracture (Fig. 12.1). The mandible, like the pelvis, is often fractured at two places, as the bone is U-shaped and is held firmly at both ends by the capsules of the temporomandibular joints.

Fractures of the *condylar* neck are caused by indirect trauma, often a blow or fall on the point of the chin, and are frequently bilateral. The detached fragment is usually angled medially and anteriorly by the pull of the lateral pterygoid muscle (Fig. 12.2).

Fractures of the *coronoid process* and *ramus* are usually caused by blunt trauma and can be difficult to detect radiographically as there may be little or no displacement at the fracture site. A fractured coronoid process (Fig. 12.3) is held in place by fibres of the temporalis muscle and a fractured ramus tends to be stabilised by the attachment of the

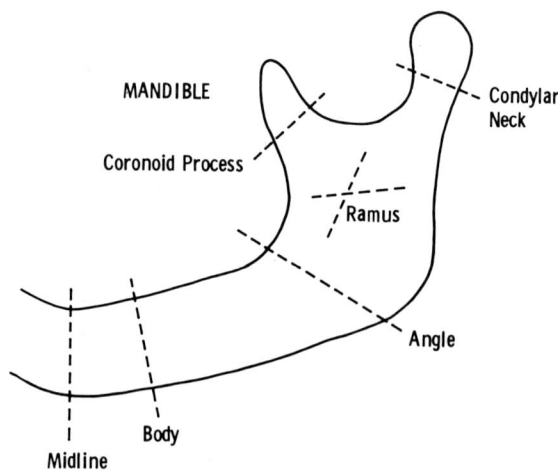

Fig. 12.1 Diagram of the common sites of fracture of the mandible.

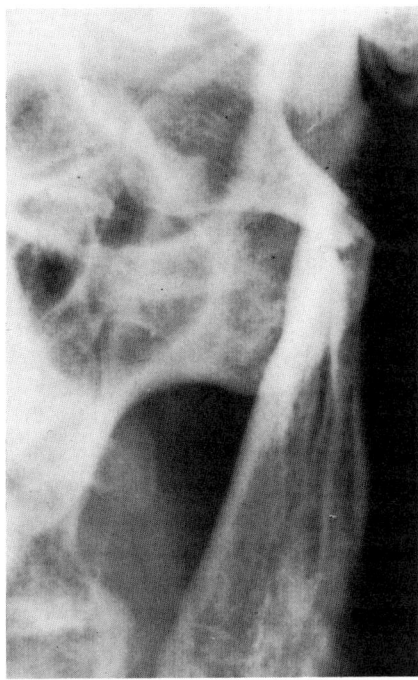

Fig. 12.2 Fracture of the condylar neck. The detached fragment is angled medially.

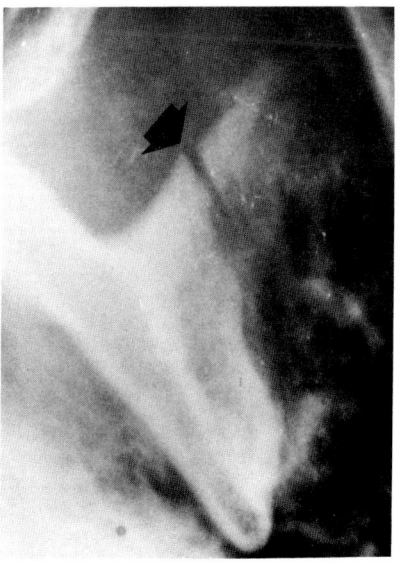

Fig. 12.3 Fracture of the coronoid process of the mandible (arrowed) on a 30° OM view.

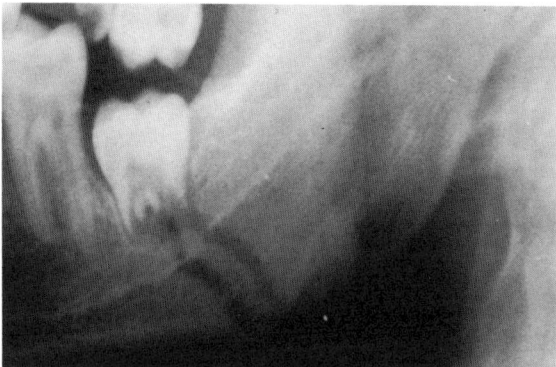

Fig. 12.4 Horizontally unfavourable fracture through the angle of the mandible. The two radiolucent lines represent fractures through the inner and outer plates. The upper end of the fracture line runs through the socket of the developing ⌐8.

masseter muscle. Fractures of the ramus are sometimes multiple or stellate.

Fractures of the *angle* and *body* are, in general, caused by direct trauma, including dental extractions. In most cases, two radiolucent lines are present on a plain radiograph as the fracture line runs obliquely and fractures the inner and outer plates at different sites (Figs 12.4, 12.5). If teeth are present the fracture line usually runs through the socket (Fig. 12.4), or even the tooth itself, as these structures are weaker than normal mandibular bone.

Fractures of the body and angle are described as *horizontally favourable* if the fracture line runs inferiorly and anteriorly (Fig. 12.5) as the muscles attached to the fragments tend to pull them together. Conversely, a fracture running posteriorly and inferiorly (Fig. 12.4) is described as horizontally unfavourable, as the fragments tend to be

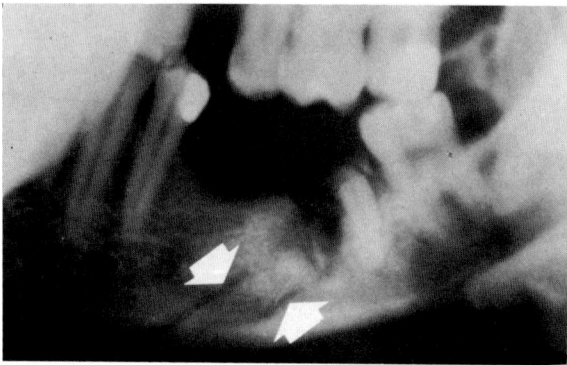

Fig. 12.5 Horizontally favourable fracture of the body of the mandible. The fracture lines through the inner and outer plates have been marked with arrows.

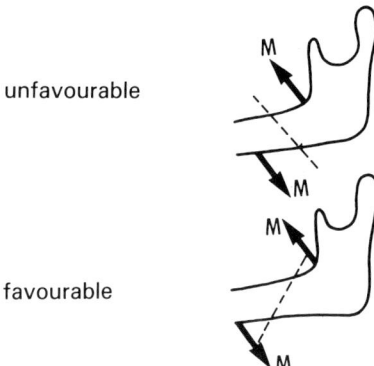

unfavourable

favourable

Fig. 12.6 Diagram of the fracture lines in horizontally favourable and unfavourable fractures of the body of the mandible. M indicates the direction of muscle pull on the anterior and posterior fragments.

pulled apart by the muscles inserted into them (Fig. 12.6). A fracture which runs anteriorly and laterally is described as *vertical favourable* as the normal muscles tone tends to approximate the fragments, whereas a fracture which runs anteriorly and medially is vertically unfavourable, as the attached muscles (mainly the medial pterygoid) tend to open the fracture by pulling the posterior fragment medially.

Most fractures of the body and angle of the mandible are compound into the mouth.

Comminuted fractures of the body and angle can result from severe trauma, usually a road traffic accident (Fig. 12.7).

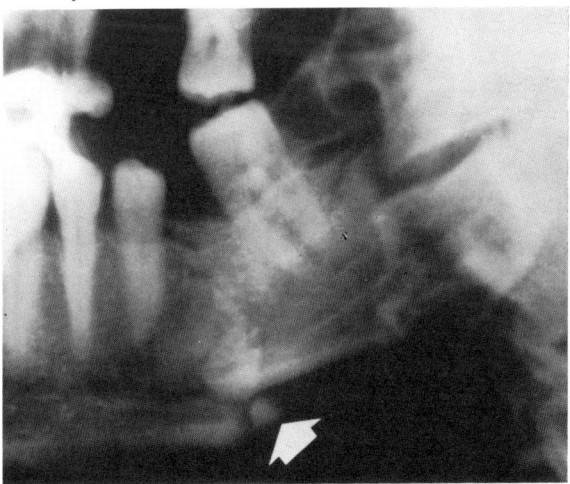

Fig. 12.7 Comminuted fracture of the body of the mandible (arrowed) with some displacement.

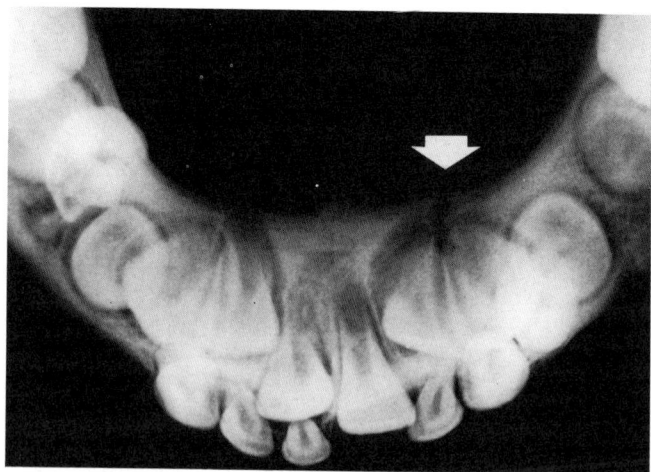

Fig. 12.8   Undisplaced fracture of the anterior part of the mandible in a child (arrowed). The fracture showed only on the intra-oral occlusal film.

Mid-line fractures and those through the anterior part of the mandible are usually caused by direct trauma and are best shown on intra-oral occlusal films. They can occur in children (Fig. 12.8) and may be comminuted if the trauma is severe (Fig. 12.9). They are usually compound into the mouth, particularly if there is any displacement.

Pathological fractures of the mandible usually affect the body and may result from infections (Fig. 8.4), cysts or tumours.

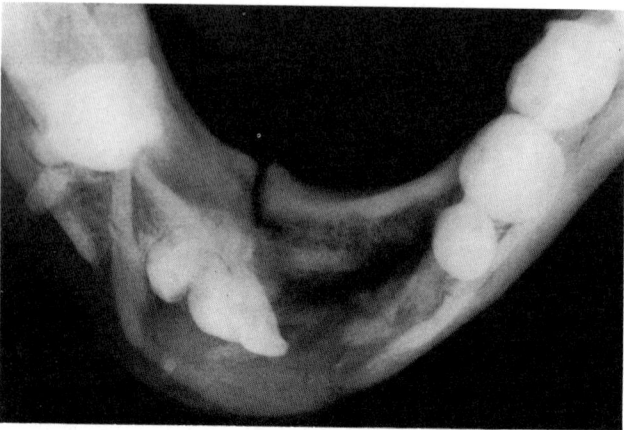

Fig. 12.9   Comminuted fracture of the anterior part of the mandible on an intra-oral occlusal film.

RADIOGRAPHIC DETECTION

Undisplaced fractures of the mandible can be difficult to demonstrate and may not show on plain films until a week after the injury, when there will be some bone resorption at the fracture site.

The initial films should consist of a PA view of the facial bones, plus oblique views of both sides of the mandible. If the patient is able to sit without support, a panoramic radiograph of the mandible should be taken, but this will not be possible if the patient has multiple injuries.

If an anterior fracture is suspected, a rotated PA film and an intra-oral occlusal film are indicated. Fractures of the condyles and condylar necks are best shown on the half-axial (Towne's) view. Fractures of the teeth and alveolar bone show most clearly on intra-oral dental films.

In some cases it will be necessary to resort to tomography of suspicious areas.

CT scanning[1] has been used to demonstrate crack fractures of the condyle and undisplaced fractures of the condylar neck, as they can be very difficult to detect on plain radiographs and even on tomograms.

REFERENCES

1. Horowitz I, Abrahami E, Mintz S S 1982 Demonstration of condylar fractures of the mandible by computed tomography. Oral Surgery, Oral Medicine, Oral Pathology 54: 263–268

13

Fractures of the maxilla

LE FORT CLASSIFICATION

Maxillary fractures are less common than mandibular fractures and are usually caused by blunt trauma. They are still classified according to the system of Le Fort, who defined three patterns of fracture, after a series of macabre experiments carried out on cadavers at the beginning of the century (Fig. 13.1).

In a *Le Fort I* fracture (Fig. 13.2) the tooth-bearing part of the maxilla become separated from the rest of the maxilla by fractures through the medial and lateral walls of the maxillary sinuses, and by a fracture through the lower part of the nasal septum.

The *Le Fort II* fracture (Fig. 13.3) is more extensive and the separated fragment is pyramidal. The apex of the pyramid is the lower part of the nasal bones and the fracture lines run inferiorly and laterally through the medial and inferior walls of the orbits and then through the lateral walls of the maxillary sinuses. The nasal septum is fractured at a variable level.

In the *Le Fort III* fracture (Fig. 13.4) there is complete cranio-facial

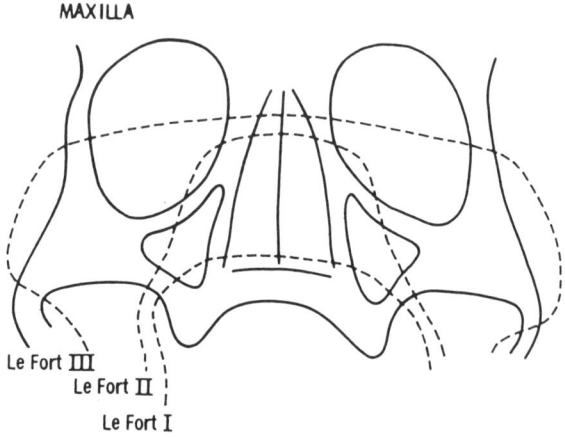

Fig. 13.1 Diagram of the fracture lines in Le Fort I, II and III fractures.

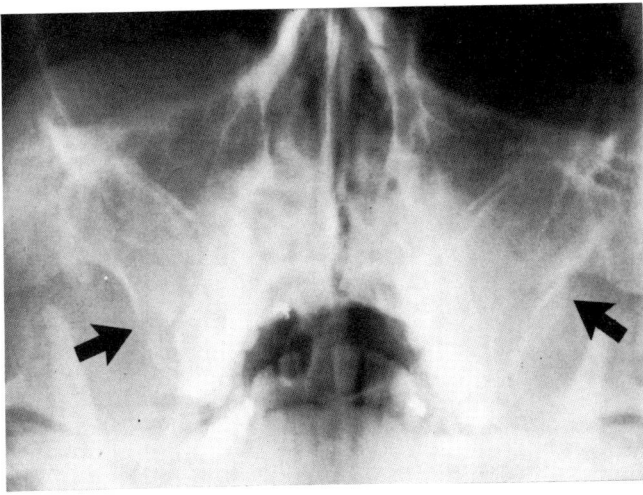

Fig. 13.2 Le Fort I fracture. The fractures of the lateral walls of the maxillary sinuses have been arrowed. The fractures of the medial walls have not been shown on this projection.

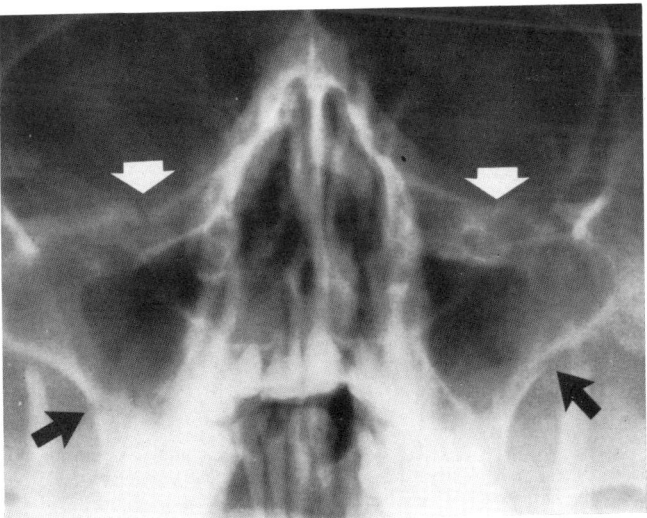

Fig. 13.3 Le Fort II fracture. The fractures of the inferior margins of the orbits and of the lateral walls of the maxillary sinuses have been arrowed. The fracture of the nasal bones is not visible on this projection.

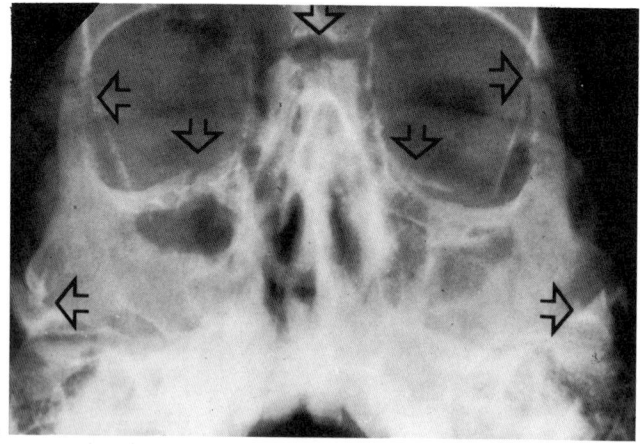

A

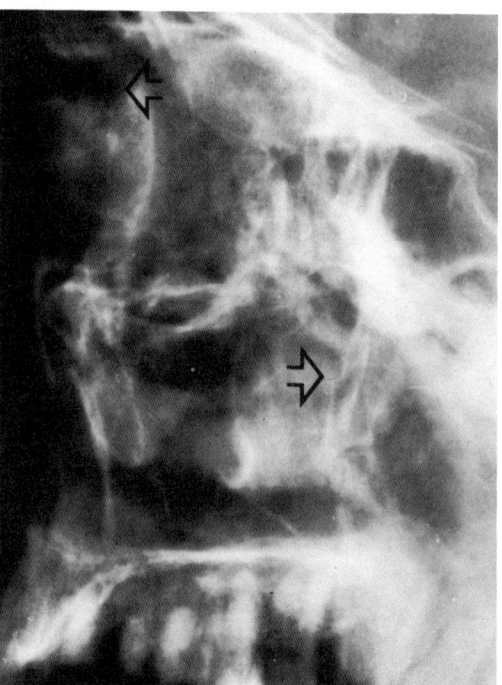

B

Fig. 13.4 A. Combined Le Fort II and Le Fort III fractures. There are fractures of the nasal bones, lateral orbital margins, inferior orbital margins and zygomatic arches (all arrowed). There is a fluid level in the right maxillary sinus and there is opacification of the left maxillary sinus. **B.** lateral view of the combined Le Fort II and III fractures shown in **A**. There is a fracture of the nasal bones with wide separation (arrowed) and there are fractures of the posterior walls of the maxillary sinuses (arrowed).

disjunction. The fracture line runs through the nasal bones as in the Le Fort II fracture, and then posteriorly and laterally through the medial and lateral walls of the orbits and through the zygomatic arches. The nasal septum is fractured superiorly.

In practice many fractures do not fit these descriptions exactly; for instance, they may be a Le Fort II fracture on one side and a Le Fort III on the other, or a Le Fort I or II fracture may co-exist with a Le Fort III (Fig. 13.4). However, the Le Fort classification is still in general use, as it allows these complicated fractures to be described in a few words, and has the additional advantage of grouping them according to the pattern of subsequent surgical management. In Le Fort I and II fractures the detached maxillary fragment is usually wired to the zygomatic arches, but if these are fractured, as in a Le Fort III fracture, it is necessary to resort to a more complicated type of pin and rod fixation to the skull vault.

Maxillary fractures due to blunt trauma are rare in *children* as the maxillary sinuses are smaller than in adults and the maxilla is relatively stronger. Severe trauma is much more likely to fracture the skull vault than the maxilla, but the penetrating trauma can result in a maxillary fracture (Fig. 13.5).

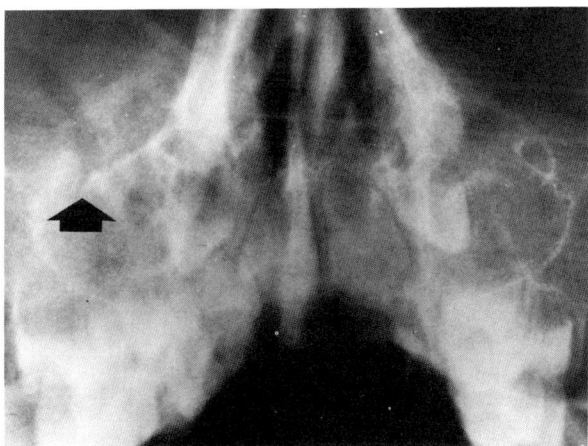

Fig. 13.5 Fracture of the right maxilla in a child with displacement at the inferior orbital margin (arrowed).

ZYGOMATIC FRACTURES

The *zygomatic bone* contributes to the lateral and inferior margins of the orbit, the lateral wall of the maxillary sinus and the anterior end of the zygomatic arch. Consequently, a fracture of the zygomatic bone results in fractures at these sites (Figs 13.6, 13.7). It is often impossible to see

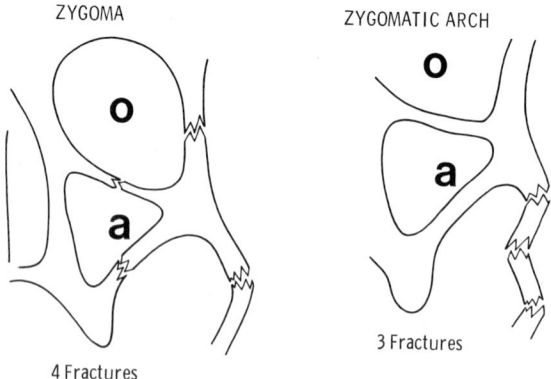

Fig. 13.6   Diagram of the usual sites of fracture of the zygoma and of the zygomatic arch. O = orbit; a = maxillary antrum.

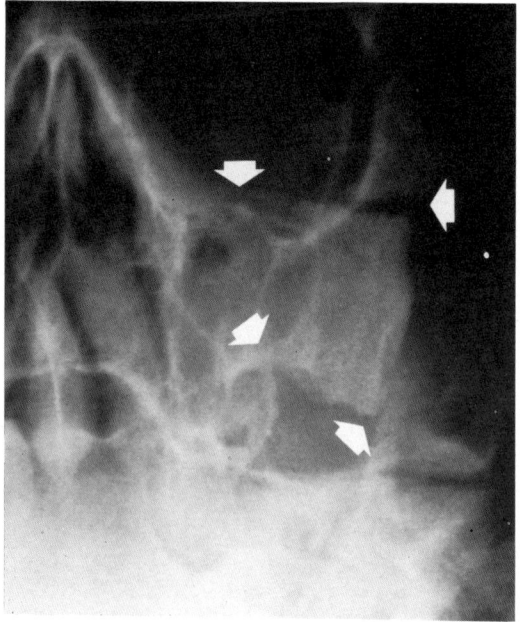

Fig. 13.7   Displaced fracture of the zygoma. The four fractures have been arrowed.

all four fractures on a single occipito–mental film, but the presence of even one fracture line should raise the suspicion of other fractures, and is an indication for further films.

The *zygomatic arch* may be fractured in association with a fracture of the zygoma as described above, or it may be fractured as a result of direct trauma, when it fractures in three places (Figs 13.6, 13.8).

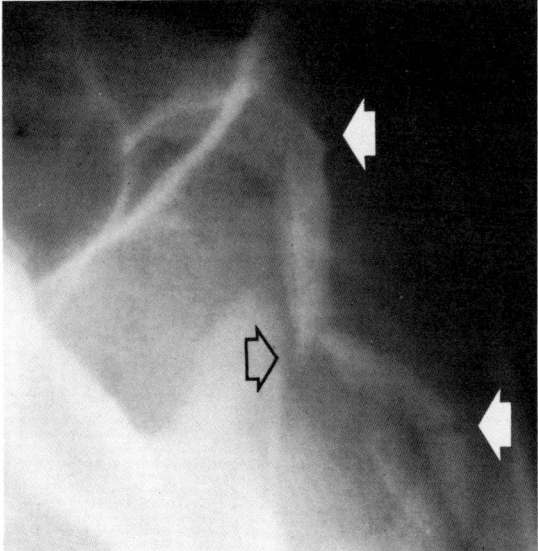

Fig. 13.8 Fracture of the zygomatic arch. The three fractures have been arrowed.

There are fractures in this region in Le Fort II and III fractures as already described.

BLOW-OUT FRACTURES

A 'blow-out' fracture of the *orbital floor* is an uncommon sequel to blunt trauma applied to the front of the orbit. The orbital rim remains intact, but the increase in pressure within the orbit causes the thin floor to fracture and the soft tissues of the orbit to herniate through the defect into the maxillary sinus.

This may show as a soft tissue shadow in the upper part of the maxillary sinus on an occipito-mental film (Fig. 13.9A), but the fractured orbital floor rarely shows on plain films. If a blow-out fracture is suspected, tomography of the orbital floor is indicated and will demonstrate a fracture if one is present (Fig. 13.9B).

The clinical importance of this fracture is that the inferior rectus and oblique muscles become attached to the orbital floor by fibrous tissue, which results in permanent limitation of upward movement of the eyeball and diplopia on looking upwards.

A blow-out fracture of the thin *lamina papyracae* of the medial wall of the orbit may occasionally follow blunt trauma to the orbit and is rarer than a blow-out fracture of the floor. The orbital contents herniate into the ethmoid sinuses in such cases.

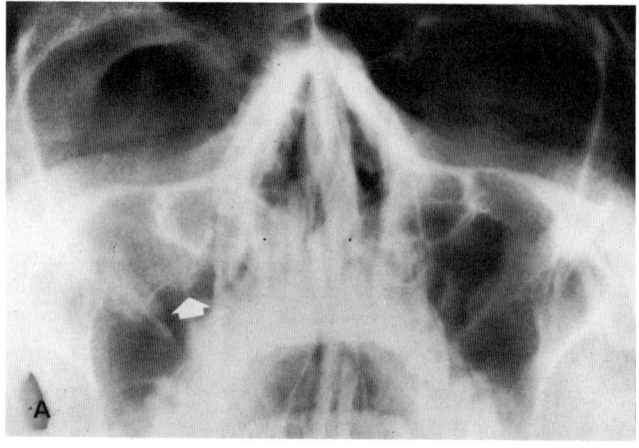

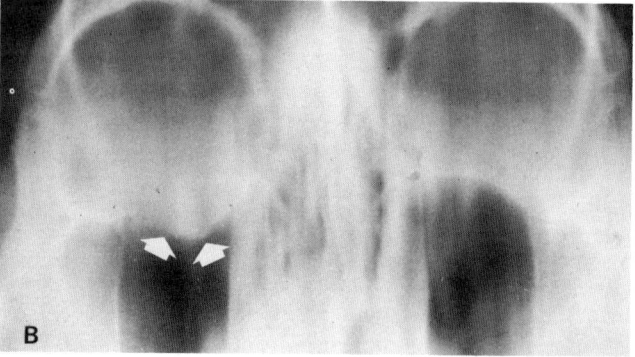

Fig. 13.9 A.   Blow-out fracture of the right orbital floor. There is soft tissue shadowing in the upper part of the right maxillary sinus (arrowed) but no fracture is visible. **B.** Tomogram of the same case, showing displaced fractures of the thin bony floor of the orbit (arrowed).

RADIOGRAPHIC DETECTION

Fractures of the maxilla and zygoma can be difficult to demonstrate radiologically, particularly if there is no displacement. The initial films should consist of an occipito–mental and a 30° occipito–mental, taken PA if possible, as this makes for better bony detail.

A lateral film of the facial bones is also useful, as it usually shows a step in the posterior wall of the maxillary sinus if the maxilla is fractured (Fig. 13.4B).

Tomography of the orbits is indicated if there is any suspicion of a blow-out fracture of the orbital floor, or if there is any indication that the orbital contents have herniated through a fracture (Fig. 13.9B).

The zygomatic arches show reasonably well on occipito–mental projections, but an underpenetrated submento–vertical view provides the clearest demonstration.

Fractures of the teeth and of the alveolar bone are best shown on intra-oral dental films.

CT scanning[1,2] has been used to diagnose maxillary fractures and is undoubtedly more accurate than plain films and tomography for undisplaced fractures and for blow-out fractures.

There are three non-specific radiological abnormalities which are often due to maxillary fractures, but which also occur in other conditions. Their presence in patients with a history of facial trauma should increase the suspicion that a fracture is present and should be an indication for further films.

1. *Soft tissue swelling* is the most common and is almost invariably present if there is a recent fracture.

2. *Opacification of the maxillary sinus* due to haemorrhage is usual if the fracture involves its wall (Le Fort I, II and III fractures, zygomatic fractures) and a fluid level is occasionally seen (Fig. 13.4A).

3. *Soft tissue emphysema* is a rare but useful sign, as it provides positive evidence of a fracture involving the nasal cavity, or one of the paranasal sinuses. It may show as multiple small radiolucent areas in the soft tissues, or air may enter the orbit to outline the eyeball (Fig. 13.10).

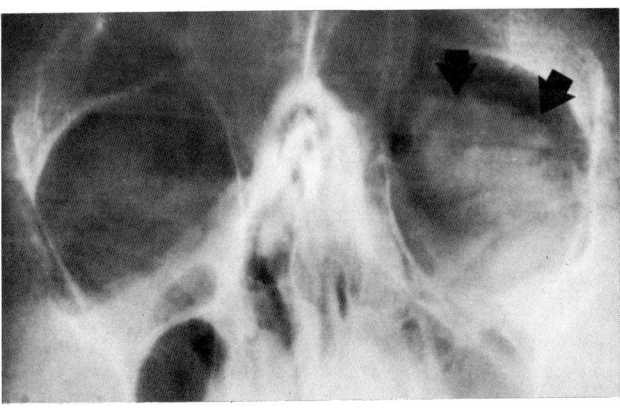

Fig. 13.10   Soft tissue emphysema of the left orbit outlining the upper margin of the eyeball. There is an undisplaced fracture of the left zygoma which cannot be identified on this film.

REFERENCES

1. Frame J W, Wake M J C 1982 Evaluation of maxillo-facial injuries by use of computerised tomography. Journal of Oral and Maxillofacial Surgery 40: 482–486
2. Kreipke D L, Moss J J, Franco J M 1984 Computed tomography and thin section tomography in facial trauma. American Journal of Roentgenology 142: 1041–1045

14

Temporomandibular joint

ANATOMY

The temporomandibular joint is a synovial joint, which is divided into upper and lower compartments by a fibrocartilagenous disc. These compartments should form separate synovial spaces and communications through the disc are always acquired abnormalities.

Two types of movement occur, firstly a hinge movement of the mandibular condyle in the glenoid fossa which takes place in the lower compartments should form separate synovial spaces and communications through the disc are usually acquired abnormalities. may pass over the maximum convexity of the articular eminence in a normal joint. The disc is attached to the mandibular condyle by the joint capsule and moves with it when the condyle moves forward.

PAIN DYSFUNCTION SYNDROME

The pain dysfunction syndrome is the clinical diagnosis most frequently applied to patients with pain in the temporomandibular joint. The condition is more common in females than in males and generally presents in early adult life.[1] The symptoms are almost invariably unilateral and tend to resolve within a year or so, even in the absence of treatment.

The aetiology is uncertain and many causes have been suggested including malocclusion, muscle spasm, stress, and internal derangement. Plain X-rays are of limited value as most symptomatic joints are radiologically normal.

Occasionally the joint space is narrowed or widened (Fig. 14.1) and the condyle may appear to be situated anteriorly or posteriorly in the glenoid fossa when the teeth are in occlusion. The detection of these minor abnormalities is largely subjective and observers often disagree about their presence or absence. The pathological significance of widening or narrowing is also uncertain and has been variously ascribed to muscle spasm, malocclusion and internal derangement.

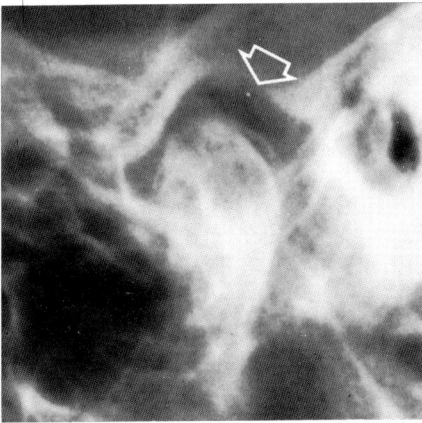

Fig. 14.1 Pain-dysfunction syndrome. The joint space is widened posteriorly (arrowed) and there is some irregularity of the anterior articular surface of the condyle.

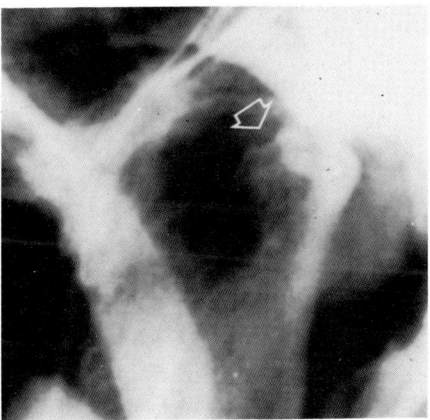

Fig. 14.2 Pain-dysfunction syndrome. A small erosion arises from the anterior aspect of the articular surface of the mandibular condyle (arrowed).

Small erosions of the anterior and superior aspects of the articular surface of the condyle are a rare feature of the pain dysfunction syndrome (Fig. 14.2). They heal gradually over a period of months and sometimes result in slight sclerosis and flattening of the antero-superior aspect of the condyle.

INTERNAL DERANGEMENT

Internal derangement should be suspected if the pain dysfunction syndrome persists for longer than a year, particularly if there are symptoms of clicking and locking.

The disc usually dislocates anteriorly and comes to lie in the anterior part of the glenoid fossa in front of the mandibular condyle. A plain film taken with the teeth in occlusion may show widening of the joint space anteriorly and a film taken with the mouth open usually shows reduced anterior movement of the condyle.

Arthrography[2,4] in these cases will show anterior extension of the inferior joint space with deformity of the superior aspect of the anterior extension due to a malpositioned disc (Fig. 14.3). This deformity usually becomes more marked on opening, but occasionally the disc

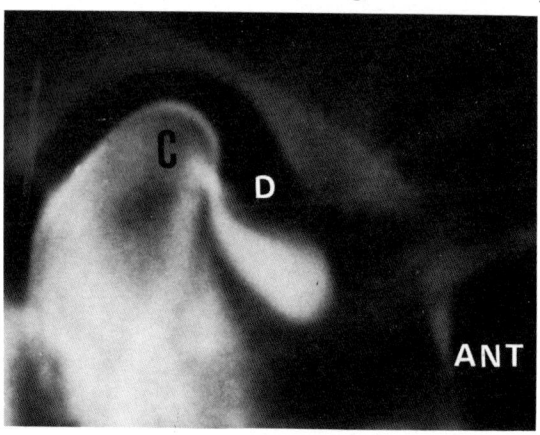

Fig. 14.3 Arthrogram showing anterior dislocation of the disc with the teeth in occlusion. The condyle C is normally situated in the glenoid fossa. The opacified inferior joint space is elongated anteriorly and deformed superiorly by the dislocated disc D.

dislocates posteriorly on opening and comes to lie behind the condyle. In these cases, arthrography will demonstrate posterior extension of the inferior joint space on opening, with deformity superiorly due to the malpositioned disc (Fig. 14.4).

Disc perforation is common in internal derangement and is readily demonstrated by arthrography, when contrast media injected into the inferior joint space will pass through the perforations into the superior compartment.[3]

OSTEOARTHRITIS

Osteoarthritis[5] (degenerative arthritis) results in the same radiological abnormalities as osteoarthritis in other synovial joints, namely narrowing sclerosis and osteophyte formation (Figs 14.5, 14.6). However, the distribution of these abnormalities is unusual, as sclerosis is confined to the mandibular condyle and osteophyte formation occurs

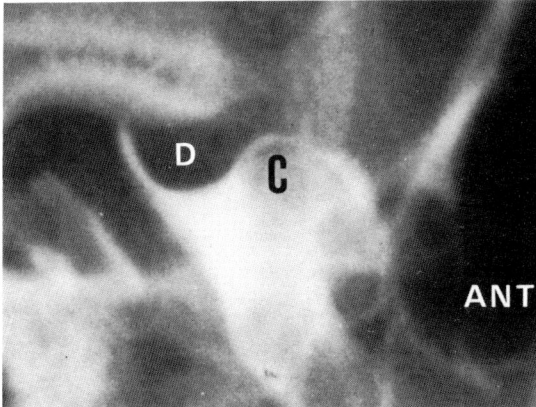

Fig. 14.4   Arthrogram showing posterior dislocation of the disc when the mouth is open. The condyle C is situated anterior to the maximum convexity of the articular eminence which is a normal appearance. The opacified inferior joint space is elongated posteriorly and deformed superiorly by the dislocated disc D.

only at the anterior aspect of the articular surface of the condyle. The glenoid fossa is always normal.

These changes are occasionally preceded by erosions of the mandibular condyle in patients with no evidence of inflammatory or infective arthritis. If the erosions are accompanied by symptoms, the patient is usually classified as suffering from the pain dysfunction syndrome, but erosions can be asymptomatic and seem to be the first radiological change of osteoarthritis in such cases.

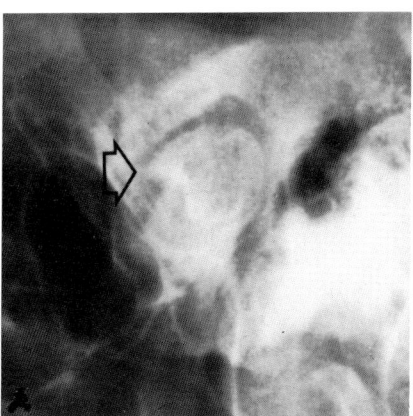

Fig. 14.5   Early osteoarthritis. There is narrowing of the joint space anteriorly with slight sclerosis. A small osteophyte arises from the anterior margin of the articular surface of the condyle (arrowed).

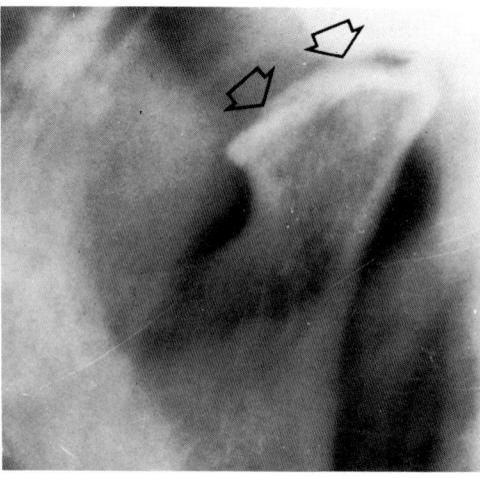

Fig. 14.6   Advanced osteoarthritis. There is flattening and sclerosis of the antero-superior aspect of the articular surface of the condyle (arrowed) and an osteophyte is present anteriorly. The width of the joint space cannot be assessed on this transpharyngeal projection taken with the mouth open.

INFLAMMATORY AND INFECTIVE ARTHRITIS

Inflammatory arthritis is a rare feature of *connective tissue diseases* such as rheumatoid arthritis, Reiter's disease and psoriasis. Erosions develop in the articular surface of the condyle and can be very extensive (Fig. 14.7). The glenoid fossa remains radiologically normal.

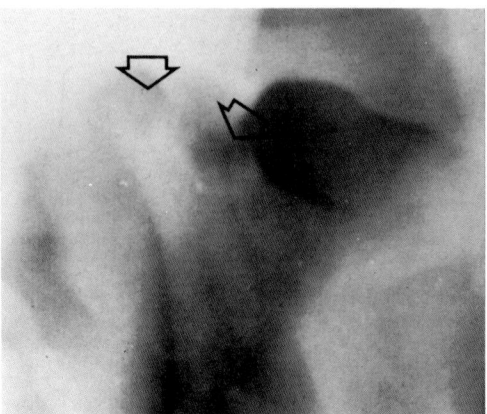

Fig. 14.7   Erosive arthritis in a patient with rheumatoid arthritis. There are large irregular erosions of the condyle and of the anterior aspect of the condylar neck (arrowed).

Infection is an even rarer cause of arthritis. It is usually due to local spread of infection from mandibular osteomyelitis or otitis externa and results in destruction of the articular surfaces of the condyle and glenoid fossa. Erosions of the mandibular condyle have been reported in patients on prolonged haemodialysis.

INJURY

Fractures of the condylar neck are common (Fig. 12.2) and rarely involve the temporomandibular joint. The condyle itself and the glenoid fossa are occasionally fractured in severe trauma, and this results in haemarthrosis.

Ankylosis of the temporo-mandibular joint may follow infective arthritis or traumatic haemarthrosis. As these disorders usually occur in childhood, most cases are complicated by hypoplasia of the mandibular condyle, due to the epiphyseal cartilage of the condylar neck having been damaged at the same time. Tomography is usually required to confirm the absence of a joint space and to demonstrate bony ankylosis between the temporal bone and the mandibular condyle (Fig. 14.8).

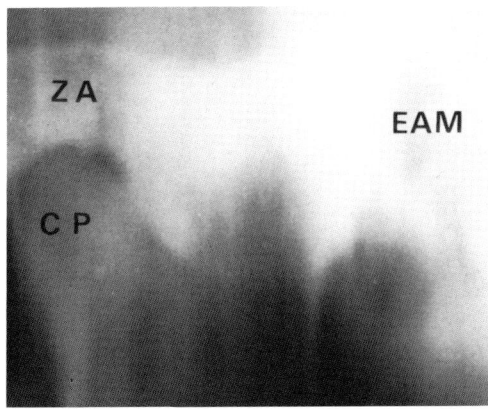

Fig. 14.8 Complete bony ankylosis of the left temporomandibular joint. The tomogram shows no evidence of a joint space. ZA = zygomatic arch. EAM = external auditory meatus. CR = coronoid process of the mandible. The patient had injured the mandible in a fall at the age of 9 years.

Dislocation of the temporo-mandibular joint is a clinical diagnosis and not a radiological one, as the condyle often moves anterior to the maximum convexity of the articular eminence in normal individuals. The role of radiology in such cases is to exclude a fracture or some other pathology such as a bone tumour.

Recurrent dislocation can be a feature of Marfan's syndrome and of the Ehlers–Danlos syndrome.

REFERENCES

1. Cawson R A 1984 Pain in the temporo-mandibular joint. British Medical Journal 288: 1857–1858
2. Doyle T 1983 Arthrotomography of the temporo-mandibular joint: a simple technique. Clinical Radiology 34: 147–151
3. Graham G S, Ferraro N F, Simms D A 1984 Perforations of the temporo-mandibular joint meniscus. Arthrographic surgical and clinical findings. Journal of Maxillofacial Surgery 42: 35–38
4. Katzberg R W, Dolwick M F, Helms C A, Mopens T, Bales D J, Coggs G C 1980 Arthrotomography of the temporo-mandibular joint. American Journal of Roentgenology 134: 995–1005
5. Kreutziger K L, Mahan P E 1975 Temporo-mandibular degenerative joint disease. Oral Surgery 40: Part I 165–182; Part II 297–319

15

Salivary glands

SIALOGRAPHY

The duct systems of the parotid and submandibular glands can be demonstrated by injecting contrast into the main duct from the mouth. The examination should always be preceded by *plain films* which will show radio-opaque calculi.

Contrast medium[2] may be oil-based (e.g. Lipiodol) or water-based (e.g. Conray 420, Urografin 370). The advantage of the more viscous oily contrast is that it remains in the duct system for a few minutes after removing the cannula and this should be long enough for the necessary films to be taken, but it has the serious disadvantage of remaining in the soft tissues for months, or even years,[1] if the duct is ruptured during cannulation, or if the injection pressure is excessive. Water-based contrast medium is safer as extravasation, although painful, is temporary. However, it is necessary to take films with the cannula still occluding the duct.

Delayed films should be taken 10 minutes after the needle or cannula has been removed, and if there is still contrast medium within the duct system it indicates duct obstruction or reduced function.

The whole gland is occasionally opacified during sialography with water-soluble or oil-based contrast medium. This appearance is known as *parenchymal opacification* and often persists after the duct system has cleared. The mechanism is uncertain, but it is probably due to reflux of contrast into the acini, with rupture and exravasation of contrast in some cases.

CALCULI

Calculi are more common in the submandibular gland than in the parotid gland and are usually a sequel to infection or stasis. Most calculi arising in the submandubular region are radio-opaque and most parotid calculi are radiolucent. Calculi are rare in children, but do occur.

Radio-opaque calculi in the submandibular duct are readily shown on intra-oral occlusal films (Fig. 15.1), and calculi within the gland itself are best shown by a lateral oblique film of the mandible, taken with the patient depressing the floor of the mouth with a finger.

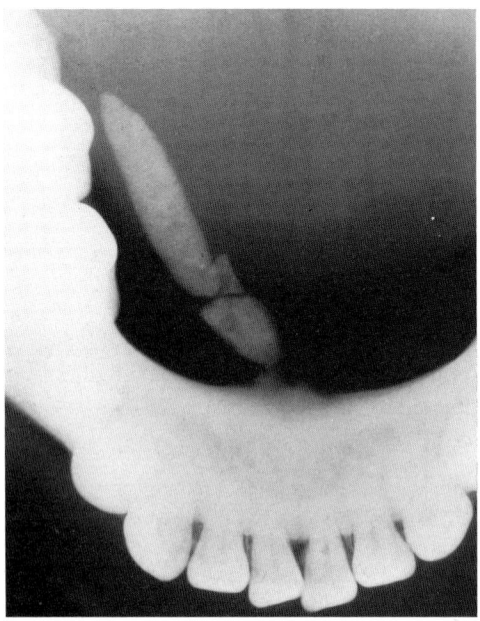

Fig. 15.1   Intra-oral occlusal view showing three radio-opaque calculi in the submandibular duct.

Radio-opaque calculi in the parotid duct or gland can usually be demonstrated on a PA film, taken if possible with the cheeks blown out (Figs 15.2, 15.3A), but small calculi situated anteriorly in the duct can only be shown on an intra-oral film which has been placed against the inside of the cheek. Radiolucent calculi can only be shown by sialography (Fig. 15.4).

Once a calculus has formed it tends to cause stasis and duct dilatation (Fig. 15.4B) which predisposes to recurrent infection, sialectasis, duct strictures (Fig. 15.5) and further calculus formation.

SIALECTASIS

Sialectasis describes a radiological appearance and simply indicates that sialography has demonstrated multiple cavities within the gland. The terms 'punctate' or 'globular' are sometimes used to describe small regular cavities measuring less than 2 mm in diameter and the term 'cavitary' to describe larger cavities with irregular walls. A cavity which exceeds 5 mm in diameter is likely to be an abscess.

Infective sialectasis can produce any of these abnormalities and is usually accompanied by calculus formation in the larger intra-glandular

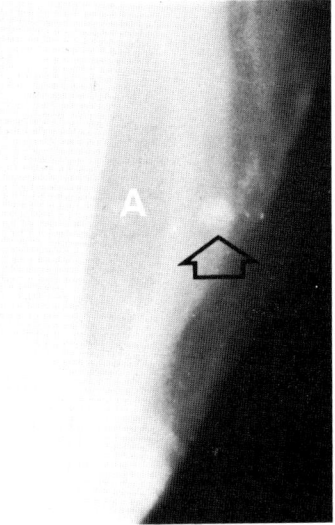

Fig. 15.2 Radio-opaque calculus (arrowed) in the lower pole of the left parotid gland on a PA film taken with the cheeks blown out. The air A in the buccal cavity shows as a radiolucent crescent medial to the soft tissues of the cheek.

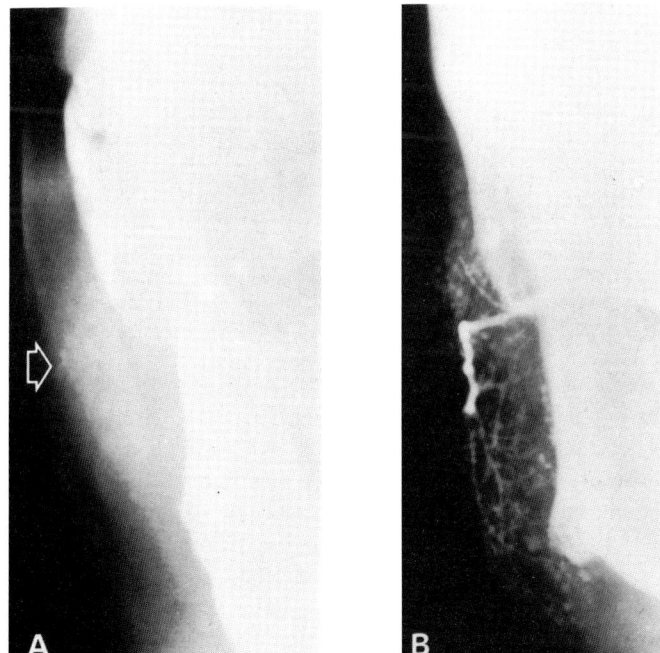

Fig. 15.3 A. Preliminary film showing multiple small calculi within the right parotid gland (arrowed). **B.** The sialogram film shows widespread sialectasis and obscures the calculi, indicating that they are situated within the sialectatic cavities. The duct system is normal.

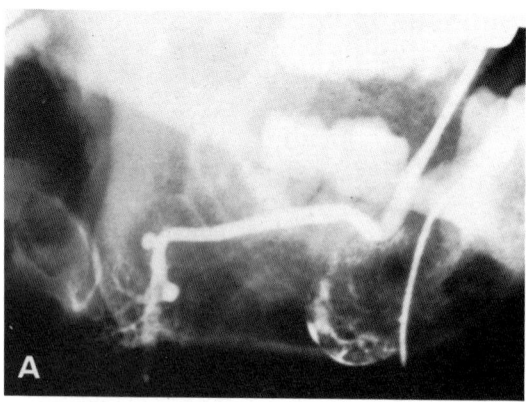

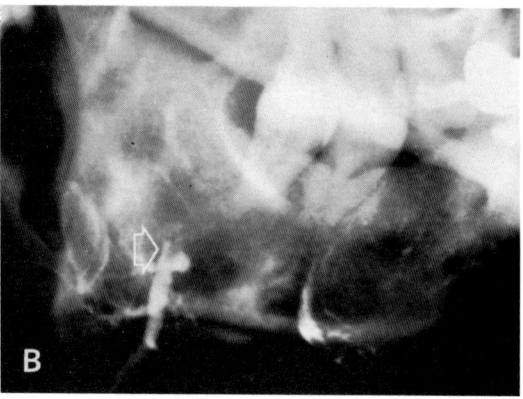

Fig. 15.4 A. Submandibular sialogram showing two sialectatic cavities in the upper part of the gland and slight dilatation of the intra-glandular ducts. **B.** Delayed film showing a small radiolucent calculus (arrowed) obstructing the main intra-glandular duct. There is slight narrowing of the duct above the calculus and generalised dilatation below.

ducts or in the main drainage duct (Fig. 15.4). Sometimes there are multiple calculi in the sialectatic cavities within the gland (Fig. 15.3).

Childhood sialectasis is a rare condition associated with intermittent tender swelling of one, or both parotid glands, which can develop at any age after 5 years and which usually resolves at puberty. It is probably due to recurrent bacterial infection and *Streptococcus* has been cultured in a few cases. However, other causes, such as virus infection, allergy and even duct obstruction, have been suggested. The term congenital sialectasis has been used to describe this condition in the past, but is rarely used now.

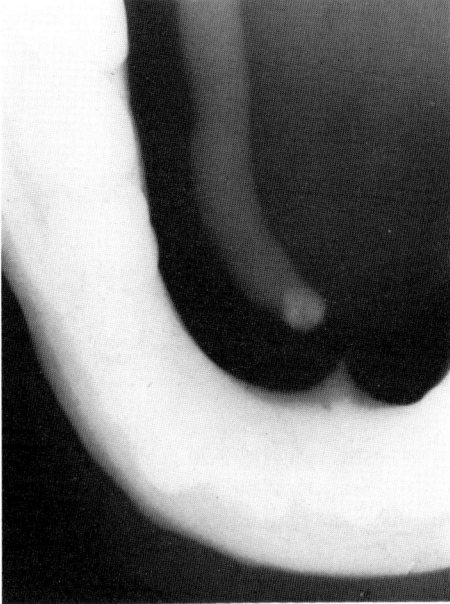

Fig. 15.5 Delayed intra-oral occlusal view taken 10 minutes after sialography showing a single radio-opaque calculus behind a stricture at the orifice of the submandibular duct.

The sialographic appearances are characteristic. There is generalised punctate sialectasis, with multiple small cavities measuring 1–2mm in diameter (Fig. 15.6). The duct system is invariably normal and there is no evidence of calculi.

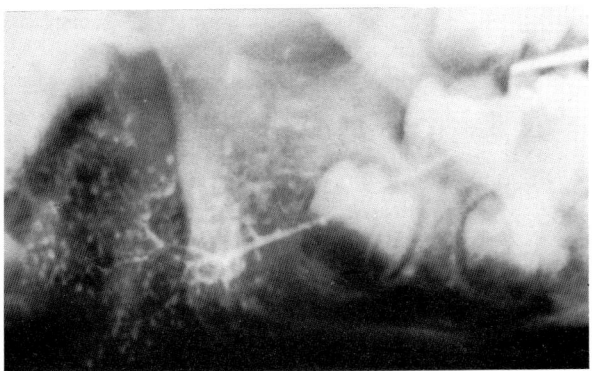

Fig. 15.6 Childhood sialectasis of the parotid gland. There is generalised punctate sialectasis with a normal duct system and no evidence of calculi.

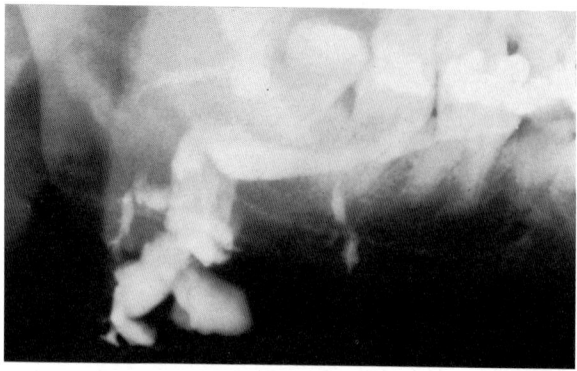

Fig. 15.7 Sjögren's syndrome. There is gross sialectasis of a submandibular gland with dilatation of the main duct.

Sjögren's syndrome and other connective tissue diseases are also associated with sialectasis. Most patients with Sjögren's syndrome have sialectasis and there is usually dilatation of the main drainage duct (Fig. 15.7).

Similar abnormalities have been described in association with a wide variety of connective tissue disorders, such as rheumatoid arthritis, systemic lupus erythematosis, ankylosing spondylitis, Reiter's disease, polyarteritis nodosa and scleroderma. The incidence of sialographic abnormalities in patients with these conditions and without any clinical evidence of Sjögren's syndrome has been estimated at 5–15%.

TUMOURS

Salivary gland tumours can develop at any age and usually present as a painless swelling. They are more common in the parotid than in the submandibular glands. The overall incidence of malignancy is 10–20%, being higher in the submandibular gland and lower in the parotid.

The typical sialographic appearance of a *benign tumour* is a duct free area within the gland, surrounded by displaced ducts which are crowded together (Fig. 15.8). If parenchymal opacification has occurred, the tumour will appear as a well defined filling defect.

Malignant tumours may have a similar appearance on sialography, but can narrow or occlude the intra-glandular ducts without displacing them and may produce an irregular parenchymal filling defect (Figs 15.9, 15.10A).

Tumours arising in the soft tissues adjacent to the parotid or submandibular glands may displace the intra-glandular ducts and produce sialographic abnormalities similar to a tumour arising in the gland itself (Fig. 15.11A).

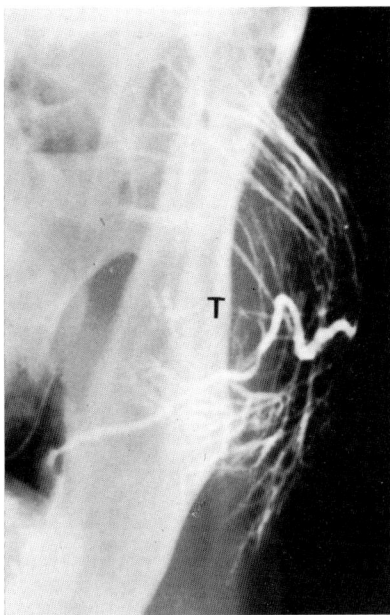

Fig. 15.8 Benign pleomorphic adenoma of the left parotid gland displacing the intra-glandular ducts but not occluding them. The site of the tumour is marked T.

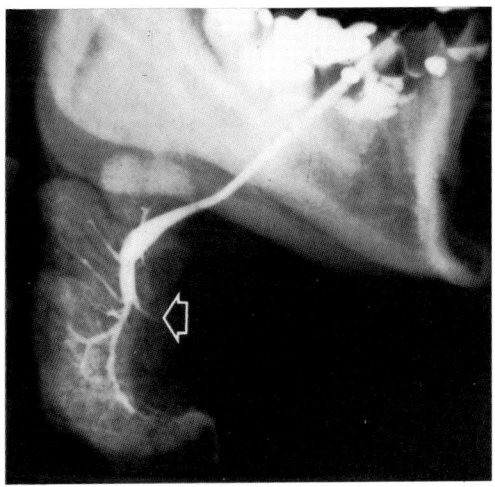

Fig. 15.9 Adenocarcinoma situated anteriorly in a submandibular gland. There is occlusion of the intra-glandular ducts in the anterior part of the gland (arrowed) and there is an irregular defect in the gland parenchyma.

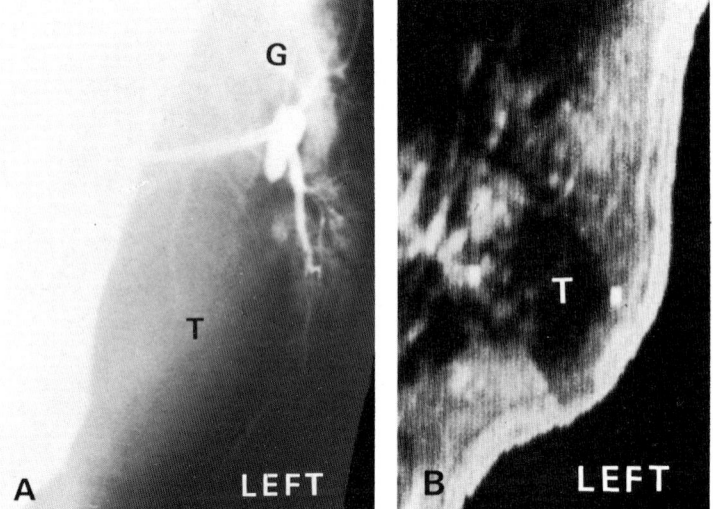

Fig. 15.10 A. Adenocarcinoma of the lower pole of the left parotid gland which has obliterated the duct system. The normal upper pole has been marked G and the tumour T. **B.** An ultrasound examination (slice in the coronal plane) shows an area of reduced echogenicity T in the lower part of the gland. The poorly defined margin is typical of an infiltrating malignant tumour.

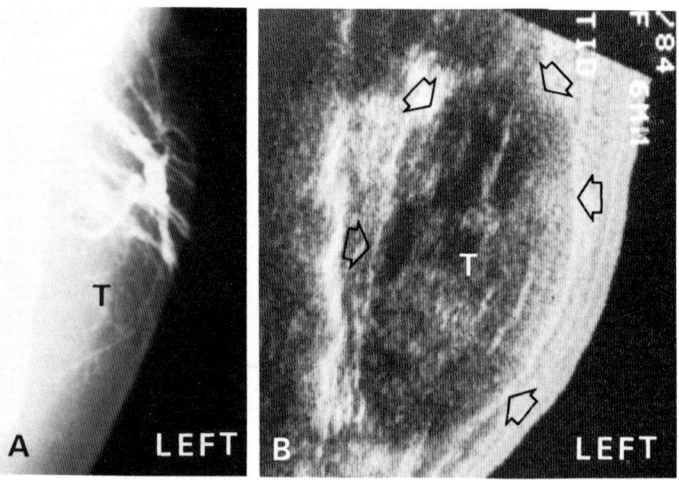

Fig. 15.11 A. Parotid sialogram showing absence of ducts in the lower part of the gland which is very suggestive of a tumour (labelled T). **B.** A coronal ultrasound scan through the gland shows a soft tissue mass T with a well defined margin (arrowed), which is typical of a benign tumour. However, the tumour is larger than the gland and extends below it. At operation, a benign neurilemmoma was found to be compressing and deforming the lower pole of the gland.

A malignant tumour arising in a palatal salivary gland may cause extensive bone destruction before it produces any symptoms.

Ultrasound is developing a useful role in the assessment of swellings in the parotid region as most lesions have a different echo pattern from the surrounding normal tissues. Solid tumours may be more or less echogenic than normal gland parenchyma, but abscesses containing pus and cysts are always relatively transonic.

Benign lesions such as tumours usually have a clearly defined margin (Fig. 15.11B), whereas malignant lesions tend to merge into the gland substance with no definite margin (Fig. 15.10B).

Isotope scanning with 1–2 mCi ^{99m}Tc pertechnetate will outline normally functioning parotid, submandibular and sublingual glands as the isotope is excreted in the saliva like iodine. Most tumours produce an area of reduced uptake, the size of which depends upon the size of the tumour. The exception is the Warthin's tumour, a rare type of benign lymphoma which concentrates the isotope and appears as an area of increased uptake or 'hot spot'.

CT scanning has been combined with sialography in the assessment of space occupying lesions within the parotid gland.[3,5] The technique will define the extent of a tumour more accurately than conventional sialography and will often distinguish between benign and malignant tumours. It is sometimes able to demonstrate the relationship of the tumour to the facial nerve.

The *pathological classification* of these tumours is complex. The benign pleomorphic adenoma is by far the most common tumour and accounts for more than half of all salivary gland tumours. Other benign tumours include papillary cystadenoma, oxyphil granular cell adenoma (oncocytoma) adenolymphoma (Warthin's tumour), adenoma and lipoma.

Malignant tumours are usually adenocarcinomas, the commonest types being muco-epidermoid carcinoma and adenoid cystic carcinoma (cylindroma). Although slow growing malignant tumours of the salivary glands have a poor prognosis and the ten year survival rate is less than 50%.

TRAUMA

Laceration of the main parotid duct, or of one of its larger intra-glandular branches, occasionally results from penetrating facial injury and is a very rare complication of surgery. Sialography will show extravasation of contrast medium from the duct system into the soft tissues (Fig. 15.12).

REFERENCES

1. Amott D G 1983 A dental radiographic artefact due to residual contrast medium. British Dental Journal 154: 331–333
2. Preece J W 1984 Choice of contrast medium sialography. Oral Surgery, Oral Medicine, Oral Pathology 57: 323–337

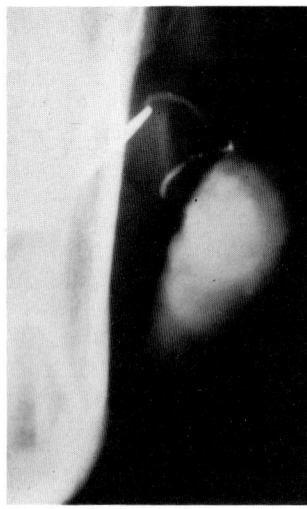

Fig. 15.12   Extravasation of contrast medium from the left parotid duct into the soft tissues. The duct had been damaged at surgery two weeks earlier.

3. Stone D N, Mancuso A A, Rice D, Hanafee W N 1981 Parotid CT sialography. Radiology 138: 393–397
4. Whaley K, Blair S, Low P S, Chisholm D M, Dick W C, Buchanan W W 1972 Sialographic abnormalities in Sjogren's syndrome, rheumatioid arthritis and other arthritides and connective tissue diseases. Clinical Radiology 13: 474–482
5. Wiesenfeld D, Ferguson M M, McMillan N C 1983 Simultaneous computed tomography and sialography of the parotid and submandibular glands. British Journal of Oral and Maxillofacial Surgery 21: 268–276

16

Soft tissues, implants and foreign bodies

SOFT TISSUE CALCIFICATION

Pulp stones can develop in the pulp chamber of any tooth and are more common posteriorly than anteriorly (Fig. 16.1). They may be a sequel to chronic inflammation, but their aetiology is uncertain. They are asymptomatic, although large stones may complicate root canal therapy.

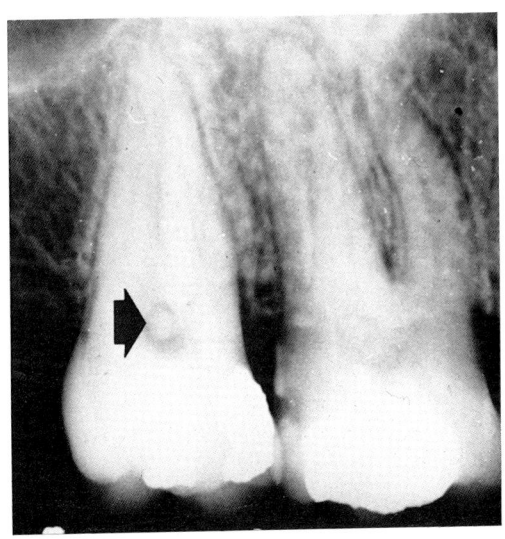

Fig. 16.1   Pulp stone (arrowed) in the pulp chamber of 8̲|.

Calcification is common in *lymphoid tissue*, especially the tonsil (Fig. 16.2) and the cervical lymph nodes and is a sequel to old infection.

Radio-opaque calculi may develop in the parotid and submandibular salivary glands and ducts (Ch. 15). Although duct calculi usually cause symptoms, calculi within the glands may be asymptomatic and are sometimes seen as an incidental radiological abnormality.

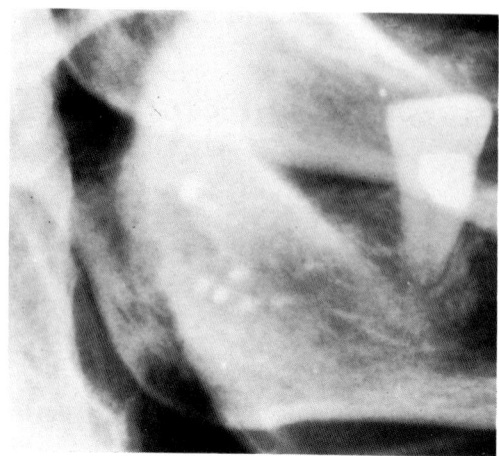

Fig. 16.2   Small areas of calcification in the tonsil.

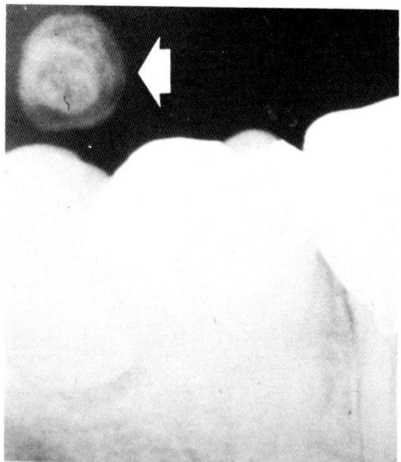

Fig. 16.3   Calcified phlebolith (arrowed) in the cheek of a young adult with a cavernous haemangioma of the face. The coencentric rings of calcification are typical.

Myositis ossificans occasionally affects the muscles of mastication. In most cases it develops in one muscle only and is precipitated by trauma, sometimes surgical. Radiologically there is calcification within the affected muscle, which is usually patchy, but which can have a linear appearance.[1] The treatment is surgical excision.

Fibrodysplasia ossificans progressiva (systemic myositis ossificans, myositis ossificans progressiva) is an extremely disabling disease of children, which results in widespread calcification of skeletal muscle. The neck muscles are affected early in the disease and the muscles of mastication are eventually affected in most cases. There is sometimes flattening of the condylar heads and shortening of the condylar necks.[3]

Calcification is occasionally seen in the walls of the facial and lingual *arteries* in patients with hypercalcaemia or renal failure.

Small ring opacities are rarely seen in the subcutaneous tissues of the face and may be due to phleboliths in a *haemangioma* (Fig. 16.3), or to multiple *miliary osteomas* of the skin.

Small areas of subcutaneous calcification have been reported in *Gorlin's syndrome* and the *Ehlers-Danlos syndrome*.

SOFT TISSUE EMPHYSEMA

Soft tissue emphysema may complicate a *maxillary fracture* (Fig. 13.10) and in most cases is precipitated by nose blowing which increases the air pressure within the nasal cavity and paranasal sinuses, forcing air into the soft tissue through a tear in the mucosal lining.

It may follow *endodontic treatment* if hydrogen peroxide is used to sterilise the root canal, or if air driven equipment is used in the mouth when the root canal is open.

Emphysema is a rare complication of *oral surgical procedures* and has been reported after *conservation treatment* with air driven equipment.

Radiologically there is an increase in the radiolucency of the affected tissues and multiple small radiolucent areas may be visible. Subcutaneous emphysema shows most clearly on an under penetrated or 'soft tissue' radiograph.

IMPLANTS

Endosseus implants (Figs 16.4, 16.5) are manufactured from chrome cobalt or titanium alloys and are densely radio-opague. When a blade or pin implant is successfully established, intra-oral radiographs will show that it is separated from normal alveolar bone by a thin radiolucent line which has been shown histologically to consist of dense connective tissue. A lamina dura sometimes develops outside the investing connective tissue.

Root resorption or localised bone rarefaction may follow insertion of a pin implant (Fig. 16.4) and is usually a bad prognostic sign, indicating eventual failure. The presence of localised bone rarefaction around a blade implant is always a bad prognostic sign and is usually due to low grade infection.

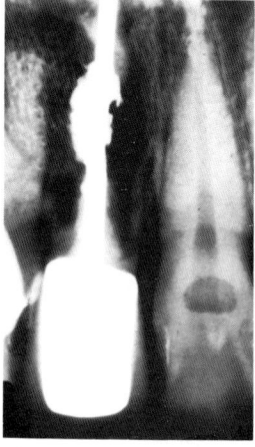
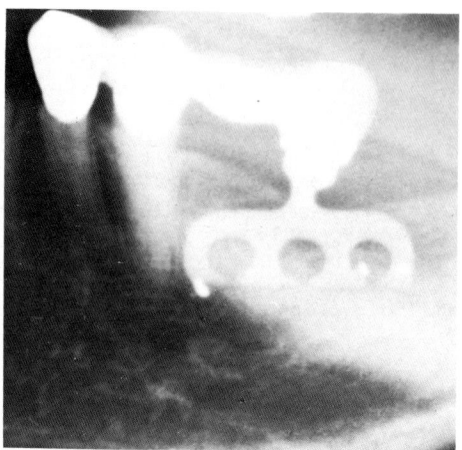

Fig. 16.4 Endosseus pin implant extending beyond the apex of ⌐1⌐ with extensive root resorption.

Fig. 16.5 Endosseus blade implant in the lower left molar area forming an abutment for a bridge.

Sub periosteal implants (Fig. 16.6) are usually cast in chrome cobalt and are densely radio-opaque. The assessment of such implants is essentially clinical, but radiographs occasionally show underlying bone rarefaction and evidence of chronic infection.

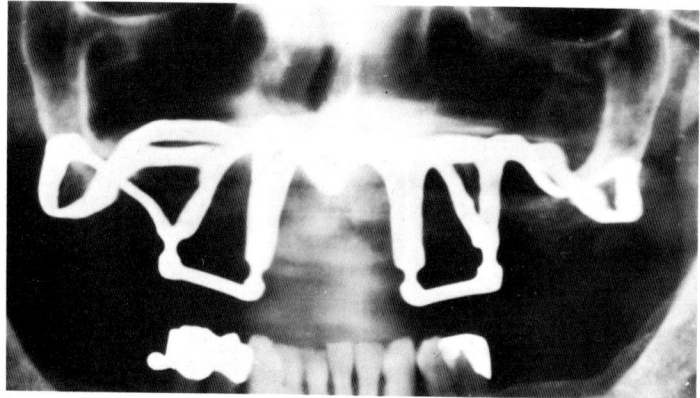

Fig. 16.6 Sub-periosteal maxillary implant.

FOREIGN BODIES

Dental amalgam (Fig. 16.7) is readily incorporated into a healing tooth socket if it is used as a filling material before the socket has developed an epithelial covering. Although the radiological abnormality can be striking, the material seems to be quite harmless and does not cause symptoms or predispose to infection.

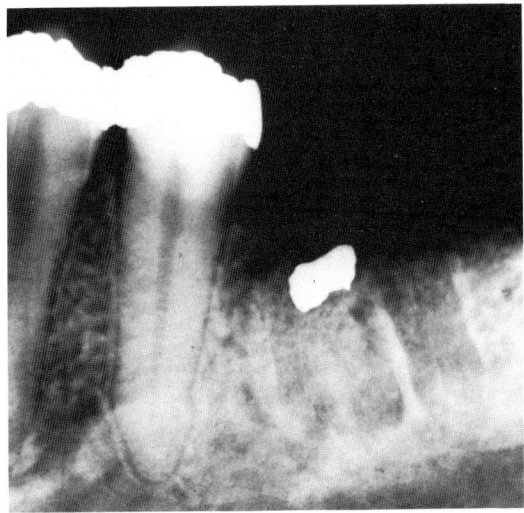

Fig. 16.7   Amalgam in a healed ⌐6 socket.

Fractured needles and *root canal instruments* show clearly as dense radio opacities (Fig. 16.8).

Lead shot, shrapnel and other *metallic missiles* in the soft tissues show clearly as they are radio-opaque (fig. 16.9).

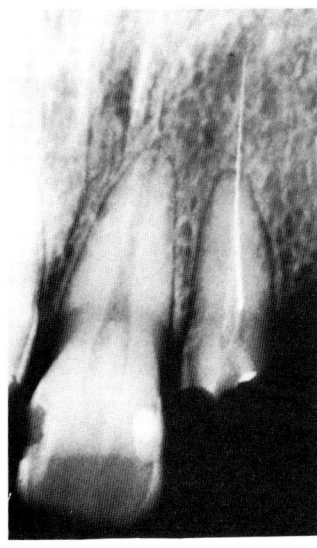

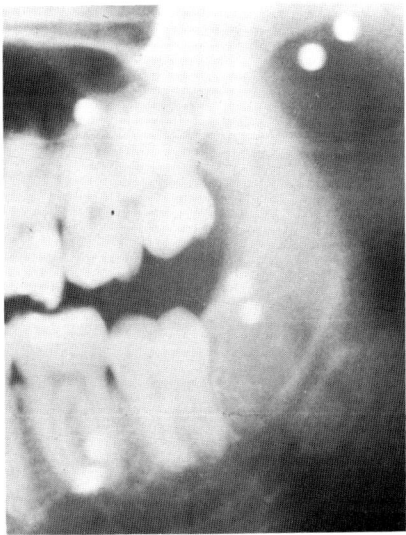

Fig. 16.8   Fractured root canal reamer extending beyond the apex of ⌊2.

Fig. 16.9   Lead shot in the soft tissues of the face.

REFERENCES

1. Christmas P I, Ferguson J W 1982 Traumatic myositis ossificans. British Journal of Oral Surgery 20: 196–199
2. Kullaan-Mikkonen A, Mikkonen M 1982 Subcutaneous emphysema. British JOurnal of Oral Surgery 20: 200–202
3. Renton P, Parkin S F, Stamp T C B 1982 Abnormal temporomandibular joints in fibrodysplasia ossificans progressiva. British Journal of Oral Surgery 20: 31–38

Appendix

Differential diagnosis of radiolucent and radio-opaque bone lesions

The following lists are not fully comprehensive, but they should make it possible to check that most diagnostic possibilities have been considered.

It should be borne in mind that they are based entirely on radiological appearances and take no account of surgical or histological findings. For instance, cysts and tumours which are radiologically multilocular usually turn out to be unilocular at operation and lesions which are completely radiolucent may contain areas of calcification when examined histologically. It should be emphasised that it is often impossible to make a precise pathological diagnosis on the radiological abnormalities alone. As in bone lesions elsewhere, the final diagnosis usually depends upon a combination of the clinical, radiological and histological features together with the appropriate biochemical and immunological tests in some cases.

Conditions which commonly produce different patterns of radiological abnormality are listed under more than one heading.

	Radiolucent	Multilocular radiolucent
COMMON	Normal dental crypt Alveolar abscess Apical granuloma Dental cyst Periodontal abscess Dentigerous cyst Nasopalatine cyst	Odontogenic keratocyst Non epithelial cyst Ameloblastoma Giant cell tumour Giant cell granuloma Dentigerous cyst
UNCOMMON	Stafne bone cavity Odontogenic keratocyst Non epithelial cyst Globulomaxillary cyst Fibrous dysplasia (early) Cementoma (early) Ossifying fibroma (early) Paget's disease (early) Pyogenic osteomyelitis Giant cell tumour Giant cell granuloma Ameloblastoma	Myxoma Dental cyst
RARE	Carcinoma Osteogenic sarcoma Myxoma Metastatic carcinoma Burkitt's lymphoma Malignant lymphoma Histocytosis X Cherubism Non pyogenic infections Hyperparathyroidism Chondroma and chondrosarcoma Haemangioma Neurofibroma, neurilemmoma Fibroma Ewing's tumour Median mandibular cyst Median palatal cyst Gumma TB osteomyelitis Midline granuloma	Haemangioma Cherubism Plasmacytoma and myeloma Metastatic carcinoma Ameloblastic sarcoma Ameloblastic carcinoma Ameloblastic fibroma Hyper parathyroidism
COMMON	Root fragment Idiopathic sclerosis (bone island) Torus mandibularis Torus palatinus Hypercementosis Supernumary tooth Supplemental tooth	Fibrous dysplasia Ossifying fibroma Cementoma

Radio opaque	Mixed radio opaque and radiolucent
UNCOMMON Fibrous dysplasia (late) Cementoma (late) Ossifying fibroma (late) Paget's disease (late) Complex composite odontome Compound composite odontome Condensing osteitis Peri-apical osteopetrosis Osteoma Osteochondroma	Compound composite odontome Chronic osteomyelitis Osteogenic sarcoma Paget's disease (early)
RARE Osteogenic sarcoma Garré's osteomyelitis Osteoradionecrosis Chronic osteomyelitis Osteochondroma Osteoid osteoma Treated metastatic carcinoma Albers-Schönberg disease Renal osteodystrophy	Calcifying epithelial odontogenic tumour of Pindborg Osteoradionecrosis Treated metastatic carcinoma Actinomycosis

FURTHER READING

Beeching B 1981 Interpreting dental radiographs. Update, London

Cohen B, Kramer I R H 1976 Scientific foundations of dentistry. Heinemann, London

Dixter C, Langlais R P, Lichty G C 1980 Paediatric radiographic interpretation. Exercises in dental radiology vol 3: Saunders, Philadelphia

Gorlin R J, Pindborg J J 1976 Syndromes of the head and neck, 2nd edn. McGraw Hill, New York

Kornblut A D, de Fries H O 1979 Malignant disease of the oral cavity. Otolaryngological Clinics of North America. Saunders, Philadelphia

Kruger G O 1979 Textbook of oral and maxillo-facial surgery. Mosby, St Louis

Langlais R B, Kasle M J 1978 Intra-oral roentgenographic interpretation. Exercises in dental radiology. Saunders, Philadelphia

Langlais R B, Bentley K C 1979 Advanced oral roentgenographic interpretation. Exercises in dental radiology 2: Saunders, Philadelphia

Lucas R B 1976 Pathology of tumours of the oral tissues, 3rd edn. Churchill Livingstone, Edinburgh

Manashil G B 1978 Clinical sialography. Thomas, Springfield, Ill

Mason D K, Chisolm D M 1975 Salivary glands in health and disease. Saunders, London

Pindborg J J, Kramer I R H 1971 Histological typing of odontogenic tumours, jaw cysts and allied lesions. WHO, Geneva

Rowe N L, Williams J L 1984 Maxillofacial injuries. Churchill Livingstone, Edinburgh

Smith N J D 1980 Dental radiography. Blackwell, Oxford

Stafne E C, Gilbilsco J A 1976 Oral roentgenographic diagnosis, 5th edn. Saunders, Philadelphia

Taybi H 1975 Radiology of syndromes. Year Book, Chicago

Trapnell D M, Bowerman J 1973 Dental manifestations of systemic disease. Butterworths, London

Wuehrmann A H, Manson-Hing L R 1977 Dental radiology, 4th edn. Mosby, St Louis

Index